AF711031

Ischemic Stroke:
From Basic Mechanisms to New Drug Development

Monographs in Clinical Neuroscience

Vol. 16

Series Editor *M. Fisher,* Worcester, Mass.

Advisory Board *L. Amaducci,* Firenze
W.G. Bradley, Miami, Fla.
H.P. Hartung, Würzburg
M.A. Moskowitz, Charlestown, Mass.

KARGER

Basel · Freiburg · Paris · London · New York ·
New Delhi · Bangkok · Singapore · Tokyo · Sydney

Ischemic Stroke: From Basic Mechanisms to New Drug Development

Volume Editor *Chung Y. Hsu*

Cerebrovascular Disease Section, Department of Neurology, Washington University School of Medicine, St. Louis, Mo.

14 figures and 5 tables, 1998

KARGER

Basel · Freiburg · Paris · London · New York · New Delhi · Bangkok · Singapore · Tokyo · Sydney

Monographs in Clinical Neuroscience

formerly 'Monographs in Neural Sciences'

Library of Congress Cataloging-in-Publication Data
Ischemic stroke: from basic mechanisms to new drug development / volume editor, Chung Y. Hsu.
(Monographs in clinical neuroscience; vol. 16)
Includes bibliographical references and index.
1. Cerebral ischemia. 2. Cerebral ischemia – Chemotherapy. I. Hsu, Chung Y. II. Series.
[DNLM: 1. Cerebral Ischemia – physiopathology. 2. Cerebral Ischemia – drug therapy. W1 MO568C v. 16 1998 / WL 355 I77 1998]
RC388.5.I83 1998
616.8′1–dc21
ISBN 3–8055–6560–7 (hard cover)

Bibliographic Indices. This publication is listed in bibliographic services, including Current Contents® and Index Medicus.

Drug Dosage. The authors and the publisher have exerted every effort to ensure that drug selection and dosage set forth in this text are in accord with current recommendations and practice at the time of publication. However, in view of ongoing research, changes in government regulations, and the constant flow of information relating to drug therapy and drug reactions, the reader is urged to check the package insert for each drug for any change in indications and dosage and for added warnings and precautions. This is particularly important when the recommended agent is a new and/or infrequently employed drug.

All rights reserved. No part of this publication may be translated into other languages, reproduced or utilized in any form or by any means electronic or mechanical, including photocopying, recording, microcopying, or by any information storage and retrieval system, without permission in writing from the publisher.

© Copyright 1998 by S. Karger AG, P.O. Box, CH–4009 Basel (Switzerland)
Printed in Switzerland on acid-free paper by Reinhardt Druck, Basel
ISBN 3–8055–6560–7

Contents

Preface

This volume on cerebral ischemia is the second in a series of monographs entitled 'Clinical Neuroscience'. The intent of this series is to survey various fields within the realm of the neurological sciences where advances in basic research are impacting upon clinical practice in a major way. There are certainly many areas in neurology and related disciplines such as neurosurgery, neuropsychology and neuroimaging where insights gained from in vitro and in vivo basic research have impacted greatly upon how patients are evaluated and managed. In this series, experts on basic clinical research will overview in a variety of neurologically related areas how enhanced basic knowledge is and will impact upon patient care. Ischemic stroke was chosen for this monograph because it is a common and devastating disorder in many countries where it is clear that understanding more about the cellular and subcellular mechanisms of ischemic injury is leading to the potential for effective therapies. Many other important topics will be surveyed in the coming years.

Until recently a generally nihilistic attitude prevailed among clinicians concerning the potential for developing therapies that would improve functional and neurological outcome after acute ischemic stroke. This did not prevent many efforts over the past 40 years to develop such a therapy. These efforts were hampered by inadequate knowledge of the basic mechanisms of focal ischemic brain injury, inadequate means to image ischemic events shortly after onset and to potentially distinguish reversibly and irreversibly injured tissue, sketchy comprehension about the individually variable nature of the therapeutic time window and clinical trial deficiencies.

It was not too long ago that acute, intravenous anticoagulation was widely employed empirically in acute ischemic stroke patients with incomplete or progressing deficits to stabilize the patient or improve outcome. There is still inadequate information to definitively evaluate this therapeutic approach, but acute anticoagulation is less commonly used currently. As knowledge about the basic events in the cascade of focal ischemic brain injury expanded, and the frequent occurrence of vascular occlusion widely recognized, therapies directed at these events have supplanted anticoagulation in clinical trials for acute ischemic stroke. This volume reviews the currently recognized important mechanisms of ischemic brain injury in detail by acknowledged experts. Understanding these mechanisms serves as the underpinning for the development of potentially effective neuroprotective therapies for acute ischemic stroke. It is likely that one or more of the therapeutic interventions directed at these mechanisms of focal ischemic brain injury will prove efficacious in currently ongoing clinical trials. Dissolving intravascular thrombi that initiate the ischemic injury cascade by impeding blood flow is an important approach to the treatment of acute ischemic stroke that is not reviewed in this volume. Tissue plasminogen activator was recently approved for the treatment of acute ischemic stroke within 3 h of onset based upon the results of an NIH-sponsored trial. Perhaps experimental stroke models and new imaging modalities such as diffusion/perfusion MRI or SPECT will help to identify how thrombolytic therapy can be best employed in the future. It is predictable that monotherapy for acute ischemic stroke, either neuroprotection or thrombolysis, will only be of limited value for improving outcome based upon our understanding of the increasingly complex nature of the mechanisms of ischemic injury. In the near future, we will begin to combine various neuroprotective therapies and thrombolysis to hopefully produce enhanced therapeutic benefits. Combination therapies should be driven by comprehension of the mechanisms of ischemic injury provided by basic research. For example, the contribution of inflammatory white blood cells and free radicals to focal ischemic injury has recently been elucidated. These mechanisms appear to be of consequence only when reperfusion occurs, implying that therapies directed against these events should be combined with successful thrombolysis and not used in isolation. Advanced imaging technology could be used to document reperfusion, before these therapies are given. The future direction of stroke research and therapeutic interventions will become more complex, but the process of ischemic injury is clearly complicated and its treatment will require the combined efforts of basic and clinical researchers to really affect outcome.

Advancement towards the elusive goal of developing effective acute ischemic stroke therapy has progressed not only in relationship to increased understanding about the mechanisms of ischemic injury, but also with increased recognition of the potential time window for intervention. If the great majority of irreversible focal ischemic injury occurred within minutes after onset, there would be little or no opportunity for therapy. A large body of experimental data, primarily derived from positron emission tomography (PET) studies, support the concept of a therapeutic window after stroke occurs during which the variety of potential interventions might improve outcome. The concept of the therapeutic window is intimately related to distinguishing a penumbral region distinct from the infarct core within the ischemic zone. Recent primate PET studies suggest that the penumbra may persist for many hours after stroke onset, particularly if good collateral flow is present. The ischemic penumbra is likely highly variable in stroke patients, leading to individual differences in the extent and duration of the therapeutic time window among stroke patients. One of the great challenges for the future in stroke research will be to provide the means to identify the penumbra in individual patients and to use this information to guide successful therapy.

Stroke patients, stroke researchers and physicians who care for stroke patients all stand on the cusp of an exciting and presumably beneficial new era. We soon will be able to rapidly evaluate and successfully treat many victims of ischemic stroke. With this volume the contributors share their knowledge and vision about how we will shortly attain these lofty goals, as painstakingly obtained experimental data leads to enhanced clinical management of acute ischemic stroke.

Marc Fisher

Mechanisms of Ischemic Brain Injury Amenable to Therapeutic Interventions

Hsu CY (ed): Ischemic Stroke: From Basic Mechanisms to New Drug Development.
Monogr Clin Neurosci. Basel, Karger, 1998, vol 16, pp 2–13

Glutamate Receptor-Mediated Neuronal Death in the Ischemic Brain[1]

Dennis W. Choi, Doug Lobner, Laura L. Dugan

Center for the Study of Nervous System Injury, Department of Neurology, Washington University School of Medicine, St. Louis, Mo., USA

Substantial evidence now indicates that the excitatory neurotransmitter, glutamate, is a key mediator of central neuronal loss consequent to hypoxic-ischemic insults [1, 2]. Brain gray matter contains millimolar levels of glutamate in large part stored inside nerve terminals. Normally, energy-dependent cellular uptake rapidly clears synaptically-released glutamate from the extracellular space. However, when tissue energy stores are compromised by hypoxia-ischemia, failure of glutamate uptake together with increased glutamate efflux can lead to a potentially toxic buildup of extracellular glutamate [3]. Furthermore, the intrinsic vulnerability of neurons to glutamate-induced neuronal death is augmented by energy depletion [4].

The idea that the toxic overstimulation of neuronal postsynaptic glutamate receptors by endogenous glutamate may contribute importantly to pathological neuronal death is not unique to hypoxic-ischemic insults. Such 'excitotoxicity' may also contribute to brain or spinal cord neuronal cell loss after several other acute insults, including hypoglycemia, prolonged seizures, and trauma [5–9]. Excitoxicity has been more speculatively linked to neuronal loss in certain chronic neurodegenerative conditions.

Glutamate Receptors

Glutamate activates four major families of receptor subtypes, three of which gate cation channels – N-methyl-*D*-aspartate (NMDA) receptors, α-

[1] Supported in part by NIH grant NS 50616.

amino-3-hydroxy-5-methylisoxazole-4-propionate (AMPA) receptors, and kainate receptors – and one of which is G-protein coupled – metabotropic glutamate receptors. The receptor populations activated by AMPA and by kainate show substantial overlap, so many investigators use the terms 'AMPA/kainate' or 'non-NMDA' receptors (although the latter is a bit ambiguous – historically, metabotropic receptors have not been included as 'non-NMDA' receptors) to refer to both receptor types together.

Nearly all mammalian central neurons are excited by application of glutamate [10]. Autoradiographic mapping has indicated that NMDA, AMPA, and kainate receptors are expressed throughout the brain [11, 12]. NMDA receptors are particularly prominent in hippocampal CA1 and in superficial layers of neocortex. AMPA receptors have a distribution generally similar to that of NMDA receptors. Kainate receptors have a distribution often complementary to that of NMDA receptors, for example high in the deeper layers of neocortex and in CA3 of hippocampus.

The channels gated by NMDA, AMPA, and kainate receptors are permeable to Na^+ and K^+ [10]. The channels opened by NMDA receptors additionally have high permeability to Ca^{2+}, whereas channels opened by AMPA or kainate receptors have variable Ca^{2+} permeability [13]. Most AMPA/kainate receptors gate channels with low Ca^{2+} permeability, and bear most of the responsibility for mediating fast excitatory synaptic currents throughout the CNS. NMDA receptors also contribute to synaptic currents, generally at later times (once the Mg^{2+} block is relieved, see below). Desensitization of AMPA/kainate receptor-mediated current may be important in terminating synaptic excitation. Desensitization of AMPA but not kainate receptors can be inhibited by benzothiadiazides [14, 15].

Under physiological conditions, ambient concentrations of Mg^{2+} attenuate current through the NMDA channel by blocking the channel in a voltage-dependent fashion [16]. However, with membrane depolarization, the Mg^{2+} block of the NMDA receptor-gated channel is relieved. Thus, if a neuron is sufficiently depolarized, it can reach a point where a regenerative NMDA receptor-mediated response can occur. The regenerative property of the NMDA receptor, together with the high Ca^{2+} permeability of its channel, likely underlie its key participation in phenomena like synaptic plasticity and epilepsy. Function of the NMDA receptor is also modified by glycine binding (required for receptor activation), extracellular pH (low pH inhibits), zinc (inhibits), redox state (oxidation inhibits), polyamines (potentiate), and phosphorylation [17].

Much information is now available about the molecular nature of glutamate receptors [18–20]. The first to be cloned were the AMPA-preferring receptors GluR-1 to GluR-4 [21] (alternatively referred to as GluR-A to GluR-D by Seeburg and colleagues). These AMPA receptor subunits – which also respond to kainate – exist in two variants, 'flip' and 'flop', achieved by alternative mRNA splicing. Flip and flop versions differ in the sequence of a 38-amino acid segment preceding the transmembrane segment nearest the C-terminal, and have distinctive electrophysiological properties; in general the flip versions allow greater net current flux. Message RNA for the flip versions is present early in developing rat brains, whereas flop mRNA starts at a low level and increases with development.

It remains to be determined exactly how individual AMPA receptor subunits are assembled to form native AMPA/kainate receptors, but it is likely that more than one subunit type, and several total subunits combine to form most native receptors. The GluR-2/GluR-B subunit – which differs from the other three AMPA receptors in having a positively charged arginine residue instead of a neutral glutamine in a critical transmembrane-spanning region – may be responsible for imparting the impermeability to Ca^{2+} and the linear I-V behavior characteristic of most (but not all) native AMPA/kainate receptor-gated channels (see below). Interestingly, this critical arginine-for-glutamine substitution likely occurs not because of DNA coding, but rather by posttranscriptional RNA editing [22].

The second major class of glutamate receptors, constituting GluR-5 to GluR-7, have high affinity for kainate but little affinity for AMPA. GluR-6 at least encodes functional kainate-activated membrane channels when expressed in oocytes. This class of glutamate receptors also contains kainate-preferring subunits, KA-1 and KA-2, which have not been demonstrated to produce functional channels in electrophysiological assays when expressed homomerically. When expressed together with GluR-5 or GluR-6, KA-2 leads to the formation of functional channels with special properties.

The third class of cloned channel-linked glutamate receptors are NMDA receptor subunits. The first NMDAR-1 receptor subunit was isolated by Nakanishi and colleagues [23], and bears 22–26% sequence homology to GluR-1. Interestingly, NMDAR-1 carries a neutral asparagine residue in the critical transmembrane-2 region corresponding to the critical, arginine/glutamine residue which governs Ca^{2+} permeability in AMPA receptors (see above). Subsequently, several related functional NMDA subtypes have been identified, named NMDAR-2A, NMDAR-2B, and NMDAR-2C; message for these have overlapping but differential expression in rat brain. The message for NMDAR-1 appears to be present in widespread fashion throughout the brain, and robust currents are elicited only when NMDAR-1 is co-expressed with one of the NMDAR-2 series receptors; these observations suggest that NMDAR-1 may be a constitutive component of native brain NMDA receptors.

The fourth class of glutamate receptors, metabotropic glutamate receptors (mGluRs), do not directly gate membrane channels, but rather act via G-proteins to alter second messenger systems [24–26]. Eight major subtypes have been cloned, classifiable by sequence and action into three groups: mGluR 1 and 5 which are positively coupled to phosphoinositol hydroloysis, mGluR 2 and 3 which are negatively coupled to adenylate cyclase, and mGluR 4, 6, 7 and 8 which are also negatively linked to adenylate cyclase but show a different agonist preference than mGluR 2/3 subtypes. Message for these different mGluRs all have distinctive distributions in brain.

Participation of Glutamate Receptors in Excitotoxicity

Different glutamate receptor subtypes do not participate equally in excitotoxicity [27]. Antagonist experiments in vitro suggest that much of the neuronal death associated with brief intense glutamate exposure requires NMDA receptor activation [28]. Glutamate-induced cortical or hippocampal neuronal death can be substantially blocked by selective blockade of NMDA receptors, although predictably (since AMPA/kainate receptors can still be activated) glutamate-induced excitation and acute neuronal swelling are only partially attenuated by the same blockade [29]. In contrast, selective blockade of AMPA/kainate receptors has only a small effect on late neuronal death. Only when both NMDA and AMPA/kainate receptors are blocked is all death, as well as acute glutamate-induced neuronal swelling, eliminated. While brief exposure to high concentrations of kainate or AMPA produce little death [30], kainate and AMPA are both highly neurotoxic if exposure time is extended for hours [29, 30]. With 24-hour exposure, low concentrations of either kainate or AMPA can kill cortical neurons [30].

Thus glutamate receptor-mediated neuronal injury, at least on cultured cortical neurons, occurs in two main patterns: (1) rapidly-triggered excitotoxicity induced by the brief intense stimulation of large numbers of NMDA receptors, and (2) slowly-triggered excitotoxicity induced by the prolonged stimulation of AMPA/kainate receptors (or the low level stimulation of NMDA receptors). The former is critically dependent on the presence of extracellular Ca^{2+}, consistent with the idea that rapidly-triggered toxicity is initiated by excessive Ca^{2+} influx through the Ca^{2+}-permeable NMDA receptor-gated channel. While measurements of average somatic intracellular free Ca^{2+} within individual neurons $[Ca^{2+}]_i$, have not revealed any simple relationship to lethal excitotoxic injury [31, 32], it remains plausible that the prominent role of NMDA receptors in neurotoxic injury reflects a special ability to move a large amount of calcium quickly into neurons [33], overloading buffering mechanisms and leading to a delayed lethal secondary rise in $[Ca^{2+}]_i$ [34].

Slowly-triggered, AMPA/kainate receptor-mediated excitotoxicity may also be initiated by excessive Ca^{2+} influx. Most channels gated directly by AMPA or kainate receptors have limited Ca^{2+} permeability, but Ca^{2+} influx can occur indirectly, for example through voltage-gated Ca^{2+} channels activated by the Na^+ influx and membrane depolarization associated with AMPA/kainate receptor stimulation. Other indirect pathways for Ca^{2+} entry may include reverse operation of the Na^+-Ca^{2+} exchanger, membrane stretch-activated conductances, or leak conductances activated by cell swelling. Perhaps longer periods of receptor stimulation are needed to induce lethal injury because the rate of Ca^{2+} influx is lower [33], and neurons may be able to cope with the influx temporarily.

In addition, some native AMPA receptors gate channels permeable to Ca^{2+} [35], as noted above, likely reflecting a molecular composition lacking the Glu-R2/Glu-RB subunit. A minority of cortical neurons, mostly inhibitory GABAergic cells, appear to possess large numbers of these AMPA receptor-gated Ca^{2+} channels, and perhaps as a direct result, are especially vulnerable to damage mediated by AMPA receptor overactivation [36–39].

Available evidence suggests that metabotropic receptor stimulation modifies, rather than mediates, excitotoxic injury. The broad-spectrum metabotropic receptor agonist, trans-1-aminocyclopentyl-1,3-dicarboxylate (trans-ACPD), is itself not directly toxic; rather, it reduces rapidly-triggered excitotoxicity [40]. This finding was at the time surprising, in view of the idea that the main effect of mGluR activation was an increase in Ca^{2+} release from intracellular stores [41, 42]. However, the recent delineation of mGluR subtypes has suggested a possible basis. Selective activation of the mGluR subtypes 1/5, which are responsible for triggering intracellular Ca^{2+} release, indeed does potentiate excitotoxic injury, whereas selective activation of the 'inhibitory' mGluRs 2/3, attenuates NMDA receptor-mediated excitotoxicity [43, 44].

Downstream Mediators of Excitotoxic Death

Glutamate neurotoxicity can be modeled as a three-stage process: induction, amplification, and expression [45]. First, the prolonged availability of extracellular glutamate is transduced by neuronal membrane receptors into potentially lethal intracellular derangements, in particular, intracellular Ca^{2+} overload. Second, modulatory events amplify these derangements, increasing their intensity and promoting the involvement of other neurons. Finally, these derangements trigger the cytotoxic cascades responsible for subsequent delayed neuronal disintegration, the expression of cell death.

It is attractive to hypothesize that abnormal movements of Ca^{2+} are the primary mediators of injury in both rapidly-triggered excitoxicity and slowly-triggered excitotoxicity. Relevant Ca^{2+} movements include in particular, the excess entry of extracellular Ca^{2+}, but may also include the release of Ca^{2+} from intracellular stores. As a result of these events, intracellular free Ca^{2+},$[Ca^{2+}]_i$, and total cellular Ca^{2+} achieve lasting elevation, eventually triggering neuronal degeneration.

Induction

As outlined above, elevated extracellular glutamate activates its array of neuronal membrane receptors, leading directly to the development of an initial set of intracellular changes – increases in cytoplasmic Ca^{2+}, Na^+, Cl^-, water, IP_3, and diacylglycerol – that serve as triggers for subsequent lethal events.

Amplification

Following the induction of glutamate toxicity, many events may potentiate resultant internal derangements, especially local elevations in $[Ca^{2+}]_i$. These amplification events may include:

(1) Additional influx of extracellular Ca^{2+} through voltage-gated Ca^{2+} channels, reverse operation of the Na^+-Ca^{2+} exchanger, Ca^{2+}-activated Ca^{2+} channels, or stretch-activated cation channels.

(2) The release of Ca^{2+} from intracellular stores, for example mediated by elevations in IP_3 [46].

(3) The activation of key enzyme families – including C kinases and clamodulin-regulated enzymes – and genes, that may act in concert to enhance processes promoting excitotoxicity, including Ca^{2+}-dependent glutamate release from nerve terminals, postsynaptic receptor responsiveness to glutamate, and Ca^{2+} influx through voltage-gated channels. The activation of phospholipase A_2 and nitric oxide synthase increases formation of the toxic intercellular messengers arachidonic acid and its eicosanoid metabolites, and nitric oxide. Once formed in postsynaptic neurons, these messengers can diffuse freely across lipid membranes to affect neighboring neurons and glia.

(4) Glutamate efflux from injured neurons, which may induce further excitotoxic injury, a positive-feedback loop that might both intensify existing injury, and help propagate excitotoxic injury onto neurons spared by the initial insult.

Expression

Sustained elevations in $[Ca^{2+}]_i$ can be expected to trigger destructive cascades capable of bearing ultimate responsibility for neuronal degeneration. Many specific Ca^{2+}-triggered destructive events may be common to rapidly-triggered excitotoxicity and slowly-triggered excitotoxicity. These include Ca^{2+}-activated catabolic enzymes, such as proteases, phospholipases, and endonucleases. Recent data suggests that the novel calpain inhibitor, MDL-28,170, has powerful protective effects against focal ischemic insults in the rodent brain, detectable even when administered up to 6 h after ischemia onset [M. Linnik, meeting commun., 1996].

A key downstream mediator of excitotoxic death is free radical formation, especially oxygen free radicals [47, 48]. Free radical production might be linked to elevated $[Ca^{2+}]_i$ in several ways, including: (1) Ca^{2+} activation of phospholipase A_2 liberating arachidonic acid which upon further metabolism leads to free radical production [49]; (2) Ca^{2+}-triggered conversion of xanthine dehydrogenase to xanthine oxidase, a rich enzymatic source of free radicals; (3) stimulation of NMDA receptors leading to the activation of nitric oxide synthase and the release of nitric oxide [50, 51] and (4) uncoupling of mitochondrial electron transport, enhancing mitochondrial production of free radicals [52, 53].

Once formed, free radicals can initiate many destructive processes including lipid peroxidation [54, 55], as well as promote further excitotoxic injury by enhancing glutamate release [56]. The topic of nitric-oxide-mediated injury is discussed further in the chapter by M. Moskowitz; the larger topic of free radical damage after brain ischemia is discussed further in the chapter by P. Chan.

Antagonizing Excitotoxicity in the Ischemic Brain

The most direct approach to blocking excitotoxic brain injury in the ischemic brain is to administer glutamate antagonist drugs. In vitro, these drugs can dramatically reduce the vulnerability of cultured neurons to deprivation of oxygen and glucose (fig. 1). Substantial evidence now suggests that NMDA antagonists can reduce infarct volume and improve functional outcome in a variety of animal stroke models [57, 58]. NMDA antagonists probably have their most important protective actions in the ischemia penumbra, an area where insult severity is submaximal, and yet NMDA receptors are probably briskly activated. A central unanswered question is how NMDA antagonists can reduce the death of nonneuronal cells, an effect implicit in infarct reduction. Is this effect secondary to reduced neuronal death, with consequent reduction of injury to cytokines or microvascular compromise?

More recent studies have suggested that AMPA/kainate antagonists may also have substantial protective effects against both global [59, 60] and focal ischemic insults [61, 62]. Possibly, the in vivo protective effects of these latter

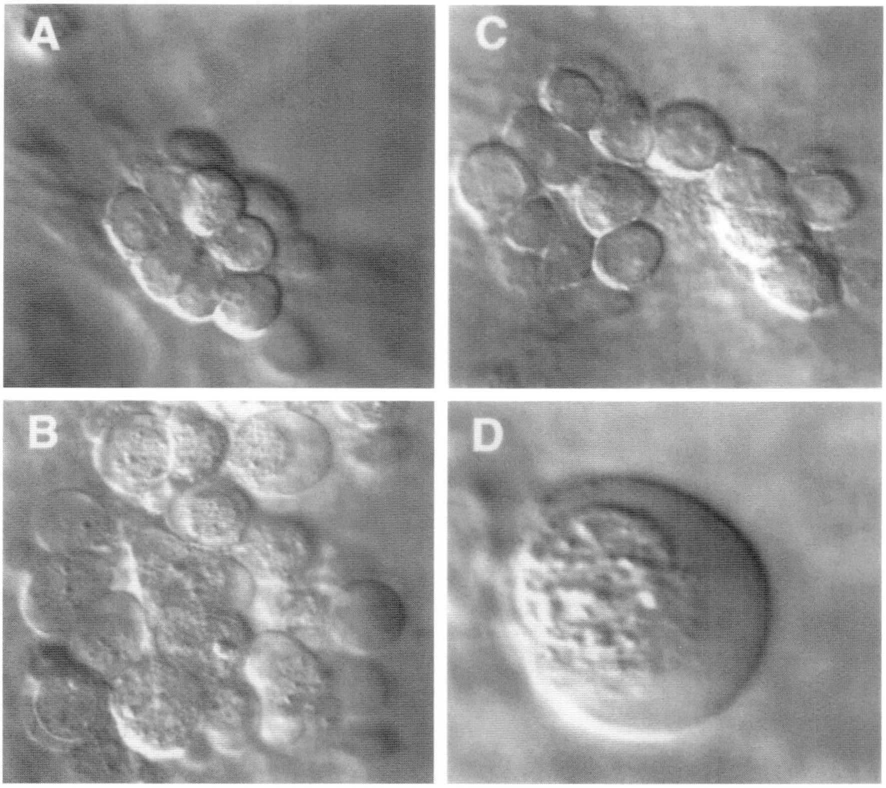

Fig. 1. Differential interference contrast photomicrographs of cultured murine cortical neurons: sham wash control (*A*), exposure for 55 min to combined oxygen-glucose deprivation either alone (*B, D*) or with 10 μM MK-801 (*C*) added during the deprivation period.

drugs reflect not only blockade of slowly-triggered AMPA/kainate receptor-mediated excitotoxicity, but also some concurrent reduction of rapidly-triggered, NMDA receptor-mediated excitotoxicity. AMPA/kainate antagonists are likely to reduce firing and depolarization in the injured brain, leading to reduction of synaptic glutamate release; they may also attenuate depolarization and carrier-mediated glutamate release from glia. In addition, the depolarization-limiting effect of these drugs may strengthen the voltage-dependent Mg^{2+} block of the NMDA receptor-gated channel directly on vulnerable neurons.

Glutamate antagonist drugs are under current development and clinical testing by several pharmaceutical companies. NMDA antagonists have potential safety risks, including acute psychotomimetic effects, disruption of synaptic plasticity, and the induction of neuronal vacuolization in a subset of neurons localized to the retrosplenial and cingulate cortices [63]. However, the first two risks are likely to be small, given acute, limited duration therapy, and an adult patient population. The risk of direct brain toxicity presents reason for pause, but the changes observed to date have been restricted anatomically, and in large part, transient and reversible. Balanced against potential substantial benefit in stroke, the unknown risks of glutamate antagonist therapy may prove to be acceptable. A major direction at present is the harnessing of cloned receptor expression systems to develop subtype-specific glutamate antagonists, with early data suggesting possible improvements in therapeutic index over broad-spectrum antagonists.

Beyond NMDA or AMPA/kainate antagonists, many other antiexcitotoxic approaches can be considered. One might block excitotoxic injury upstream of postsynaptic glutamate receptors, for example by inhibiting glutamate release (adenosine agonists, hypothermia, Na^+ channel blockers, N- or P-type Ca^{2+} channel blockers), or downstream of postsynaptic receptors by blocking some of the cytotoxic consequences triggered by receptor overactivation. mGluR agonists at the 'inhibitory' subtypes, mGluR 2 and mGluR 3, may limit excitotoxicity (see above) by reducing Ca^{2+} influx through voltage-gated channels and glutamate release from presynaptic terminals. Blockers of voltage-gated sodium or calcium channels might help limit intracellular cation overload.

In another chapter, M. Linnik discusses emerging evidence that some of the cell death induced by hypoxia-ischemia may occur via intrinsic cell death mechanisms involved in normal developmental cell death. This 'ischemic apoptosis' is likely substantially distinct from ischemic excitotoxicity, and thus antiapoptosis strategies may be additive to antiexcitotoxic strategies. My colleagues and I have found that the combination of the NMDA antagonist, dextrorphan, and the protein synthesis inhibitor, cycloheximide, can produce a dramatic reduction of infarct volume after focal ischemia in rats, greater than that achievable with either drug alone [64].

References

1 Simon RP, Swan JH, Griffiths T, Meldrum BS: Blockade of N-methyl-*D*-aspartate receptors may protect against ischemic damage in the brain. Science 1984;226:850–852.

2 Choi DW, Rothman SM: The role of glutamate neurotoxicity in hypoxic-ischemic neuronal death. Annu Rev Neurosci 1990;13:171–182.

3 Benveniste H, Drejer J, Schousboe A, Diemer NH: Elevation of the extracellular concentrations of glutamate and aspartate in rat hippocampus during transient cerebral ischemia monitored by intracerebral microdialysis. J Neurochem 1984;43:1369–1374.

4 Novelli A, Reilly JA, Lysko PG, Henneberry RC: Glutamate becomes neurotoxic via the N-methyl-*D*-aspartate receptor when intracellular energy levels are reduced. Brain Res 1988;451:205–212.
5 Wieloch T: Hypoglycemia-induced neuronal damage prevented by an N-methyl-*D*-aspartate antagonist. Science 1985;230:681–683.
6 Meldrum B: Possible therapeutic applications of antagonists of excitatory amino acid neurotransmitters. Clin Sci 1985;68:113–122.
7 Olney JW, Collins RC, Sloviter RS: Excitotoxic mechanisms of epileptic brain damage. Adv Neurol 1986;44:857–877.
8 Faden AI, Demediuk P, Panter SS, Vink R: The role of excitatory amino acids and NMDA receptors in brain injury. Science 1989;244:798–800.
9 Hayes RL, Jenkins LW, Lyeth BG, Balster RL, Robinson SE, Clifton GL, Stubbins JF, Young HF: Pretreatment with phencyclidine, and N-methyl-*D*-aspartate antagonist, attenuates long-term behavioral deficits in the rat produced by traumatic brain injury. J Neurotrauma 1988;5:259–274.
10 Mayer ML, Westbrook GL: The physiology of excitatory amino acids in the vertebrate central nervous system. Prog Neurobiol 1987;28:197–276.
11 Monaghan DT, Holets VR, Toy DW, Cotman CW: Anatomical distributions of four pharmacologically distinct ^{3}H-*L*-glutamate binding sites. Nature 1983;306:176–179.
12 Greenamyre JT, Young AB, Penney JB: Quantitative autoradiographic distribution of *L*-[^{3}H]glutamate-binding sites in rat central nervous system. J. Neurosci 1984;4:2133–2144.
13 Macdermott AB, Dale N: Receptors, ion channels and synaptic potentials underlying the integrative actions of excitatory amino acids. Trends Neurosci 1987;10:280–284.
14 Yamada KA, Tang CM: Benzothiadiazides inhibit rapid glutamate receptor desensitization and enhance glutamatergic synaptic currents. J Neurosci 1993;13:3904–3915.
15 Partin KM, Patneau DK, Winters CA, Mayer ML, Buonanno A: Selective modulation of desensitization at AMPA versus kainate receptors by cyclothiazide and concanavalin A. Neuron 1993;11:1069–1082.
16 Ascher P, Nowak L: Electrophysiological studies of NMDA receptors. Trends Neurosci 1987;10:284–288.
17 McBain CJ, Mayer ML: N-methyl-*D*-aspartic acid receptor structure and function. Physiol Rev 1994;74:723–760.
18 Seeburg PH: The TINS/TIPS Lecture. The molecular biology of mammalian glutamate receptor channels (review). Trends Neurosci 1993;16:359–365.
19 Hollmann M, Heinemann S: Cloned glutamate receptors. Annu Rev Neurosci 1994;17:31–108.
20 Nakanishi S: The molecular diversity of glutamate receptors (review). Prog Clin Biol Res 1994;390:85–98.
21 Hollmann M, O'Shea-Greenfield A, Rogers SW, Heinemann S: Cloning by functional expression of a member of the glutamate receptor family. Nature 1989;342:643–648.
22 Seeburg PH: The role of RNA editing in controlling glutamate receptor channel properties (review). J Neurochem 1996;66:1–5.
23 Moriyoshi K, Masu M, Ishii T, Shigemoto R, Mizuno N, Nakanishi S: Molecular cloning and characterization of the rat NMDA receptor (see comments). Nature 1991;354:31–37.
24 Nakanishi S: Molecular diversity of glutamate receptors and implications for brain function. Science 1992;258:597–603.
25 Scheopp DD, Conn PJ: Metabotropic glutamate receptors in brain function and pathology. Trends Pharmacol Sci 1993;14:13–20.
26 Pin JP, Duvoisin R: The metabotropic glutamate receptors: Structure and functions (review). Neuropharmacology 1995;34:1–26.
27 Choi DW: Excitotoxic cell death. J Neurobiol 1992;23:1261–1276.
28 Choi DW, Koh J, Peters S: Pharmacology of glutamate neurotoxicity in cortical cell culture: Attenuation by NMDA antagonists. J Neurosci 1988;8:185–196.
29 Frandsen A, Drejer J, Schouboe A: Direct evidence that excitotoxicity in cultured neurons is mediated via N-methyl-*D*-aspartate (NMDA) as well as non-NMDA receptors. J Neurochem 1989;53:297–299.
30 Koh J, Goldberg MP, Hartley DM, Choi dW: Non-NMDA receptor-mediated neurotoxicity in cortical culture. J Neurosci 1990;10:693–705.

31 Michaels RL, Rothman SM: Glutamate neurotoxicity in vitro: Antagonist pharmacology and intracellular calcium concentrations. J Neurosci 1990;10:283–292.

32 Tymianski M, Charlton MP, Carlen PL, Tator CH: Source specificity of early calcium neurotoxicity in cultured embryonic spinal neurons. J Neurosci 1993;13:2085–2104.

33 Hartley DM, Choi DW: Delayed rescue of N-methyl-*D*-aspartate receptor-mediated neuronal injury in cortical culture. J Pharmacol Exp Ther 1989;250:752–758.

34 Randall RD, Thayer SA: Glutamate-induced calcium transient triggers delayed calcium overload and neurotoxicity in rat hippocampal neurons. J Neurosci 1992;12:1882–1895.

35 Iino M, Ozawa S, Tsuzuki K: Permeation of calcium through excitatory amino acid receptor channels in cultured rat hippocampal neurons. J Physiol 1990;424:151–165.

36 Yin H, Turetsky D, Choi DW, Weiss JH: Cortical neurons with Ca^{2+} permeable AMPA/kainate channels display distinct receptor immunoreactivity are GABAergic. Neurbiol Dis 1994;1:43–49.

37 Turetsky D, Canzoniero LMT, Sensi SL, Weiss JH, Goldberg MP, Choi DW: Cortical neurons exhibiting kainate-activated Ca^{2+} uptake are selectively vulnerable to AMPA/kainate receptor-mediated toxicity. Neurbiol Dis 1994;1:101–110.

38 Brorson JR, Manzolillo PA, Miller RJ: Ca^{2+} entry via AMPA/KA receptors and excitotoxicity in cultured cerebellar Purkinje cells. J Neurosci 1994;14:187–197.

39 Geiger JRP, Melcher T, Koh D-S, Sakmann B, Seeburg PH, Jonas P, Monyer H: Relative abundance of subunit mRNAs determines gating and Ca^{2+} permeability of AMPA receptors in principal neurons and interneurons in rat CNS. Neuron 1995;15:193–204.

40 Koh JY, Palmer E, Cotman CW: Activation of the metabotropic glutamate receptor attenuates N-methyl-*D*-aspartate neurotoxicity in cortical cultures. Proc Natl Acad Sci USA 1991;88:9431–9435.

41 Nicoletti F, Wroblewski JT, Novelli A, Alho H, Guidotti A, Costa E: The activation of inositol phospholipid metabolism as a signal-transducing system for excitatory amino acids in primary cultures of cerebellar granule cells. J Neurosci 1986;6:1905–1911.

42 Sugiyama H, Ito I, Hirono C: A new type of glutamate receptor linked to inositol phospholipid metabolism. Nature 1987;325:531–533.

43 Bruno V, Copani A, Battaglia G, Rafaele R, Shinozaki H, Nicoletti F: Protective effect of the metabotropic glutamate receptor agonist, DCG-IV, against excitotoxic neuronal death. Eur J Pharmacol 1994;256:109–112.

44 Buisson A, Choi DW: The inhibitory mGluR agonist, S-4-carboxy-3-hydroxy-phenylglycine selectively attenuates NMDA neurotoxicity and oxygen-glucose deprivation-induced neuronal death. Neuropharmacology 1995;34:1081–1087.

45 Choi DW: Methods for antagonizing glutamate neurotoxicity. Cerebrovasc Brain Metab Rev 1990; 2:105–147.

46 Mody I, MacDonald JF: NMDA receptor-dependent excitotoxicity: The role of intracellular Ca^{2+} release. Trends Pharmacol Sci 1995;16:356–359.

47 Dykens JA, Stern A, Trenker E: Mechanism of kainate toxicity to cerebellar neurons in vitro is analogous to reperfusion tissue injury. J Neurochem 1987;49:1222–1228.

48 Monyer H, Hartley DM, Choi DW: 21-Aminosteroids attenuate excitotoxic neuronal injury in cortical cell cultures. Neuron 1990;5:121–126.

49 Chan PH, Fishman RA, Longar S, Chen S, Yu A: Cellular and molecular effects of polyunsaturated fatty acids in brain ischemia and injury; in Kogure K, Hossmann K, Siesjo B, Welsh F (eds): Progress in Brain Research. Amsterdam, Elsevier Science, 1985, vol 63, pp 227–235.

50 Garthwaite J: Glutamate, nitric oxide and cell-cell signalling in the nervous system. Trends Neurosci 1991;14:60–67.

51 Dawson VL, Dawson TM, London ED, Bredt DS, Snyder SH: Nitric oxide mediates glutamate neurotoxicity in primary cortical cultures. Proc Natl Acad Sci USA 1991;88:6368–6371.

52 Reynolds IJ, Hastings TG: Glutamate induces the production of reactive oxygen species in cultured forebrain neurons following NMDA receptor activation. J Neurosci 1995;15:3318–3327.

53 Dugan LL, Sensi SL, Canzoniero LMT, Handran SD, Rothman SM, Lin T-S, Goldberg MP, Choi DW: Mitochondrial production of reactive oxygen species in cortical neurons following exposure to N-methyl-*D*-aspartate. J Neurosci 1995;15:6377–6388.

54 Braughler JM, Hall ED: Central nervous system trauma and stroke. I. Biochemical considerations for oxygen radical formation and lipid peroxidation. Free Radic Biol Med 1989;6:289–301.
55 Seisjo BK, Agardh CD, Bengtsson F: Free radicals andd brain damage. Cerebrovasc Brain Metab Rev 1989;1:165–211.
56 Pellegrini-Giampietro DE, Cherici G, Alesiani M, Carla V, Moroni F: Excitatory amino acid release from rat hippocampal slices as a consequence of free-radical formation. J Neurochem 1988;51: 1960–1963.
57 Albers GW, Goldberg MP, Choi DW: N-methyl-*D*-aspartate antagonists: Ready for clinical trial in brain ischemia? Ann Neurol 1989;25:398–403.
58 Buchan AM: Do NMDA antagonists protect against cerebral ischemia: Are clinical trials warranted? Cerebrovasc Brain Metab Rev 1990;2:1–26.
59 Sheardown M, Nielsen E, Hansen A, Jacobsen P, Honore T: 2,3-Dihydroxy-6-nitro-7-sulfamoyl-benzo(F)quinoxaline: A neuroprotectant for cerebral ischemia. Science 1990;247:571–574.
60 Diemer NH, Jorgensen MB, Johansen FF, Sheardown M, Honore T: Protection against ischemic hippocampal CA1 damage in the rat with a new non-NMDA antagonist, NBQX. Acta Neurol Scand 1992;86:45–49.
61 Buchan AM, Xue D, Huang ZG, Smith KH, Lesiuk H: Delayed AMPA receptor blockade reduces cerebral infarction induced by focal ischemia. Neuroreport 1991;2:473–476.
62 Smith SE, Meldrum BS: Cerebroprotective effect of a non-methyl-*D*-aspartate antagonist, GYKI 52466, after focal ischemia in the rat. Stroke 1992;23:861–864.
63 Olney JW, Labruyere J, Price MT: Pathological changes induced in cerebrocortical neurons by phencyclidine and related drugs. Science 1989;244:1360–1362.
64 Du C, Hu R, Csernansky CA, Liu XZ, Hsu CY, Choi DW: Additive neuroprotective effects of dextrorphan and cycloheximide in rats subjected to transient focal cerebral ischemia. Brain Res 1996;718:233–236.

Dennis W. Choi, Center for the Study of Nervous System Injury, Department of Neurology,
Box 8111, Washington University School of Medicine, 660 S. Euclid Avenue,
St. Louis, MO 63110 (USA)

Hsu CY (ed): Ischemic Stroke: From Basic Mechanisms to New Drug Development.
Monogr Clin Neurosci. Basel, Karger, 1998, vol 16, pp 14–27

Oxygen Radical Mechanisms in Cerebral Ischemia and Reperfusion

Pak H. Chan

Departments of Neurological Surgery and Neurology, University of California School of Medicine, San Francisco, Calif., USA

Oxygen free radicals or oxidants have been implicated in the development of many neurological disorders and brain dysfunctions [1–6]. A role that oxygen free radicals may play in brain injury appears to involve reperfusion after cerebral ischemia. In either global or focal cerebral ischemia, cerebral blood flow (CBF) is significantly reduced in the brain regions that are supplied with oxygen by the occluded vessel. Reoxygenation during reperfusion provides oxygen to sustain neuronal viability and also provides oxygen as a substrate for numerous enzymatic oxidation reactions that produce reactive oxidants. In addition, reflow following occlusion often causes an increase in oxygen to levels that cannot be utilized by mitochondria under normal physiological flow conditions (fig.1). It has been demonstrated that about 2–5% of the electron flow in isolated brain mitochondria produces superoxide ($O_2{\bullet}^-$) and hydrogen (H_2O_2) [7]. These constantly produced oxygen radicals are scavenged respectively by superoxide dismutases (SODs) and by glutathione peroxidases, and catalase. Other antioxidants, including gluthathione, ascorbic acid, and vitamin E are also likely to be involved in the detoxification of free radicals. During reperfusion, it is likely that these antioxidative defense mechanisms are perturbed as a result of the overproduction of oxygen radicals, inactivation of detoxification systems, consumption of antioxidants, and the failure to adequately replenish them in the ischemic brain tissue. Due to technical difficulties, the level of oxygen free radicals in brain tissue following ischemia is generally assessed by indirect methods, including lipid peroxidation [8, 9], protein oxidation [10], and DNA damage [11, 12] (fig. 1). Recent advances in methodologies have allowed investigators to measure hydroxyl radicals by salicylate hydroxylation [13] and NO• radicals by a porphyrinic microsensor

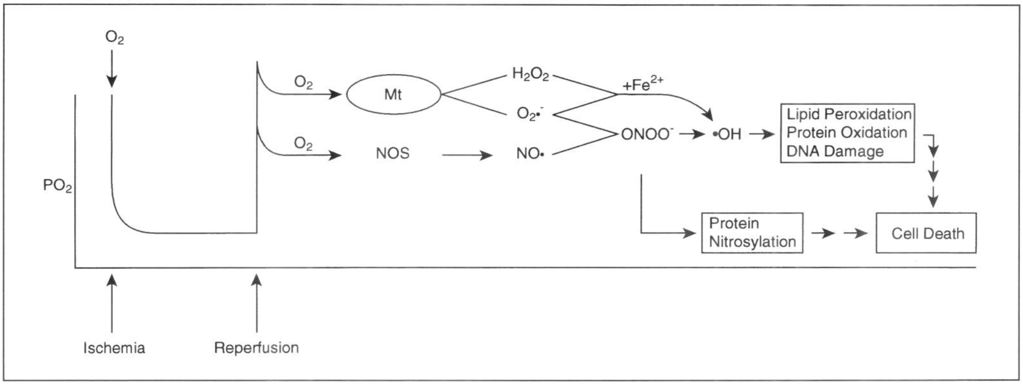

Fig. 1. Oxygen radicals in cerebral ischemia and reperfusion injury. NOS = Nitric oxide synthase; $O_2•^-$ = superoxide radicals; Mt = mitochondria; NO• = nitric oxide; •OH = hydroxyl radicals; $ONOO^-$ = peroxynitrite; H_2O_2 = hydrogen peroxide; Fe^{2+} = ferrous iron.

[14] and by electron paramagnetic resonance spin trapping [15] in ischemic brain tissue. In addition, several chemical and biochemical methods have been developed to measure superoxide radicals in neurons that undergo oxidative stress [16–20]. Despite these useful measurements for $O_2•^-$, hydroxyl (•OH) and NO• radicals, establishment of the causative role of oxygen radicals in ischemic brain injury remains a difficult task for stroke researchers and neuroscientists. This chapter will review the role of oxygen radicals in cerebral ischemia and the molecular genetic approaches employing transgenic and knockout mutant mice to dissect out the molecular and cellular mechanisms involving oxygen radicals in ischemic brain damage.

Oxygen Radical Production in Ischemic Brain

Several oxygen radical species which include $O_2•^-$, perhydroxyl ($HO_2•$), H_2O_2, and •OH, are formed following the initial reduction of oxygen:

$$O_2 + e^- \rightarrow O_2•^- \quad (1)$$
$$O_2•^- + H^+ \rightarrow HO_2• \quad (2)$$
$$O_2•^- + O_2•^- \xrightarrow{+2H^+} H_2O_2 \quad (3)$$
$$H_2O_2 \rightarrow H_2O + O_2 \quad (4)$$

In equation 3, SOD catalyzes this reaction at physiological pH at an extremely fast, constant rate (2×10^9 l mol^{-1}), forming H_2O_2 which is then detoxified to H_2O and O_2 by catalase in mammalian cells or in the brain by glutathione peroxidase (GSHPx) at the expense of reduced glutathione (GSH) (equation 4). The oxidized glutathione can be recycled to GSH by glutathione reductase in the presence of nicotinamide-adenine dinucleotide phosphate.

Hydroxyl radicals (•OH) are extremely active oxidants. These radicals are known to initiate lipid peroxidation and to cause protein oxidation and DNA damage in cells. Superoxide radicals ($O_2 {\bullet}^-$), on the other hand, are much less reactive, but have a longer half-life and can form •OH through a Haber-Weiss reaction (see equation 5):

$$O_2{\bullet}^- + H_2O_2 \rightarrow {\bullet}OH + OH^- + O_2 \qquad (5)$$
$$O_2{\bullet}^- + NO{\bullet} \rightarrow ONOO^- \qquad (6)$$
$$ONOO^- + H^+ \rightarrow ONOOH \qquad (7)$$
$$ONOOH \rightarrow {\bullet}OH + NO_2{\bullet} \qquad (8)$$

It is generally believed that this reaction (equation 5) can only proceed in the presence of trace metal iron (Fenton reaction). Another pathway for forming •OH radicals is through the reaction of $O_2{\bullet}^-$ and NO•, a gas radical that is constantly being formed in the brain neuronal, endothelial, and glial nitric oxide synthases [21, 22]. The product of this reaction is peroxynitrite ($ONOO^-$) [23].

This reaction (equation 6) is quite rapid, since the constant rate of $ONOO^-$ formation (6.7×10^9 1 mol^{-1} s^{-1}) is closed to the constant rate for diffusion [24]. At neutral pH, $ONOO^-$ degrades instantly to •OH and nitrogen dioxide ($NO_2{\bullet}$) (see equation 8). $ONOO^-$, a stronger pro-oxidant, can react with SOD to form a powerful nitrating agent resulting in the nitration of tyrosines of cellular proteins (fig.1) [25]. However, the role of $ONOO^-$ in ischemic brain injury has only recently been investigated. On the other hand, contradictory reports have surfaced with regard to the role of NO• in ischemic neuronal injury, primarily due to its dual role as vasodilator (i.e., increases in CBF) [26–31] and as a free radical that can injure neuronal cells [32–34]. Recent studies have suggested that the redox state of NO• may determine its role as either neuronal protector or injurious mediator following activation of N-methyl-*D*-aspartate receptors [35, 36]. It is of interest to note that downregulation of CuZn-SOD activity in PC12 cells by exposure to antisense oligonucleotides leads to apoptotic cell death via the NO•–$ONOO^-$ pathway [37].

Antioxidant Enzyme SODs and Cerebral Ischemia

Several enzymes, including SOD, GSHPx, glutathione reductase and catalase are endogenous antioxidants that process specific free radical scavenging properties. SODs, in particular, have been used extensively to reduce superoxide radical-associated ischemic brain damage (table 1).

Table 1. Mammalian SODs

	CuZn-SOD	Mn-SOD	EC-SOD
Location	cytosol	mitochondria	extracellular space
MW	32,000	88,000	120,000
Structure	dimer	tetramer	tetramer
Metals (g-atoms/subunit)	Cu 1, Zn 1	Mn 1	Cu 1, Zn 1
KSOD, $M^{-1}s^{-1}$	1.2×10^9	1.3×10^9	1×10^9
Chromosome	21 (human)	6 (human)	?
	17 (mouse)	16 (mouse)	?
Gene designation	*SOD*-1	*SOD*-2	*SOD*-3
Disease	amyotrophic lateral sclerosis (familial)	?	?

SOD = Superoxide dismutase; MW = molecular weight (in kilodaltons).

Based on the metal ion requirements and the anatomical distribution, three types of SODs exist in brain cells. CuZn-SOD is a cytosolic enzyme that requires both copper and zinc ions as co-factors. It is a dimeric protein that is coded by the human CuZn-SOD transgene (*SOD*-1) on chromosome 21 in human cells. Manganese (Mn-SOD) is a mitochondrial enzyme with requirements for Mn^{2+} [38]. It is a tetrameric protein that is coded by the *SOD*-2 gene in chromosome 4 in human cells. Both CuZn-SOD and Mn-SOD from various sources have been fully characterized biochemically and the cDNAs of both human enzymes have been successfully cloned [39, 40]. A copper-containing SOD (*sod*-3) has been identified in the extracellular space and its gene successfully cloned (table 1) [41]. As specified, for superoxide radicals, CuZn-SOD has been used extensively to reduce brain injury induced by ischemia and reperfusion. Unfortunately, investigators have obtained varying degrees of success and failure when free, nonmodified SOD was used to ameliorate ischemic brain injury (table 2) [58]. The extremely short half-life of CuZn-SOD (6 min) in circulating blood and its failure to pass the blood-brain barrier (BBB) make it difficult to employ enzyme therapy in cerebral ischemia. However, a modified enzyme with an increased half-life, such as polyethylene glycol-conjugated SOD (PEG-SOD), has been successfully used to reduce infarct volume in rats that have been subjected to focal cerebral ischemia [45, 57]. Liposome-entrapped SOD has an increased half-life (4.2 h), BBB permeability, and cellular uptake, and it has also proven to be an effective treatment in reducing the severity of traumatic and focal ischemic brain injuries [47, 59]. Yet, in some instances, modified SOD (i.e., PEG-SOD) has been

Table 2. Role of exogenous SOD on cerebral ischemia

Study	Animal species	SOD	Effects	Ref.
Cardiac arrest	dogs	free + deferoxamine	+	42
Complete cerebral ischemia	dogs	free + free catalase	–	43
Global cerebral ischemia	rats	free	+	44
Focal cerebral ischemia	rats	PEG	+	45
Ischemia/reperfusion	gerbils	free	+	46
Focal cerebral ischemia	rats	liposome	+	47
2-V + hypotension	rats	free	–	48
Bilateral MCA occlusion	gerbils	pyran	+	49
Global ischemia/reperfusion	piglets	PEG	–	50
Ischemia/reperfusion	dogs	liposome	+	51
Global ischemia/reperfusion	gerbils	human recombinant	+	46
Cerebral ischemia	piglets	PEG	+	52
Cerebral ischemia/reperfusion	gerbils	endogenous induction	+	53
Focal cerebral ischemia/reperfusion	rabbits	free	+	54
Global cerebral ischemia	dogs	derivative (albumin bound)	+	55
Hypoxic ischemia	piglets	PEG	–	56
Focal cerebral ischemia/reperfusion	rats	PEG	+	57

SOD = Superoxide dismutase; PEG = polyethylene glycol; MCA = middle cerebral artery.

used with conflicting results [58]. The fact that the results are mixed make it imperative to emply other experimental strategies so that the role of SOD can be fully established in cerebral ischemia.

Transgenic and Knockout Mutant Mice as Useful Tools to Study the Role of Oxidants in Ischemic Brain Injury

One strategy is to employ transgenic (Tg)/knockout technology to alter the levels of pro-oxidants, antioxidants and oxidant-related enzymes or proteins and to study the role of a specific antioxidant in ischemic brain injury.

The most commonly used method for creating Tg mice is the microinjection of DNA of interest (transgene) into the pronuclei of fertilized mouse oocytes [60]. This technique is used to introduce a linear DNA fragment (genomic or cDNA with proper promoter) which contains sequences required for directing correct transcriptional initiation and for encoding a gene product (protein, enzyme) that can be readily identified using various biochemical assays. Pronuclear microinjection of DNA leads to random integration of various copies of injected DNA into a single site on a mouse chromosome. The integrated DNA can be passed on to future generations. Another way to produce Tg mice is to introduce foreign genes to embryonic stem cells (ES) [61]. The Es cells are subsequently screened for the integration of transgenes. These ES cells with the transgene (active or inactive knockout) can then be microinjected into the blastocytes to further produce chimeric mice. The mating of chimeric mice with wild-types produces heterozygous offspring (+/−) that contain the transgene. Further, breeding among heterozygous mice generates homozygous animals (+/+ for overexpression, −/− for knockout). Using this Tg technology, several mice strains with various genotypes that relate to oxidant/antioxidant enzymes/proteins have been successfully developed. Most of these Tg and knockout mutant animals have been used in the study of the role of oxidants in ischemic brain injury (table 3).

In the studies employing Tg mice overexpressing *SOD*-1, two models of focal cerebral ischemia are used. One model is achieved by permanent occlusion of the left middle cerebral artery (MCA) just proximal to the pyriform branch of the anesthetized mouse. Immediately following occlusion of the MCA, the left common carotid artery (CCA) is permanently ligated and the right CCA is temporarily occluded for 1 h followed by additional reperfusion for 24 h. The total infarct volume (mm^3) is reduced by 36% in *SOD*-1 Tg mice as compared to non-transgenic (nTg) mice. The brain edema is also reduced in both the MCA territory and the anterior cerebral artery area, a region that corresponds to the 'ischemic penumbra'. Antioxidants, both GSH and ascorbic acid, are maintained at higher levels in the penumbra area than in the same anatomical regions in nTg mouse brains [75]. In another study that involved the use of *SOD*-1 Tg mice, MCA occlusion is achieved with a 5-0 rounded nylon suture placed within the internal cerebral artery followed by withdrawal of the suture to allow reperfusion. The infarct volume is reduced by 26% in *SOD*-1 Tg mice at 3 h of reperfusion after 3 h of ischemia [63] and by 40% in *SOD*-1 Tg mice at 24 h after 1 h of MCA occlusion, as compared to nTg mice (fig. 2) [76]. The decrease in the infarct volume in *SOD*-1 Tg mice clearly parallels the reduction of neurological deficits and is not related to the changes in CBF. On the other hand, infarct volume produced in *SOD*-1 Tg mice that are subjected to 24 h of permanent MCA occlusion using intraluminal suture blockade is not different from that of nTg mice [64] suggesting that the increased ischemic severity resulting from prolonged cerebral ischemia will limit the protective role of CuZn-SOD against neuronal injury.

In addition to the *SOD*-1 Tg mice, Tg mice overexpressing basic fibroblast growth factor (bFGF), when subjected to right CCA ligation, hyperglycemia and 20 min of 1% carbon monoxide, contained more viable hippocampal CA neurons than nTg mice [66]. Although the mechanism by which the bFGF

Table 3. Transgenic and knockout mutant mice in the study of the role of oxidants in ischemic brain surgery

Gene	Enzyme/Protein	Transgene/knockout	Study	Effect	Ref.
SOD-1	CuZn-superoxide dismutase	human transgene	focal cerebral ischemia	+	62
SOD-1	CuZn-superoxide dismutase	human transgene	transient focal cerebral ischemia	+	63
SOD-1	CuZn-superoxide dismutase	human transgene	permanent focal cerebral ischemia	NP	64
BCL-2	BCL-2 protein	human transgene neuronal-specific	Permanent focal cerebral ischemia	+	65
bFGF	Basic fibroblast growth factor	human transgene	hypoxia/ischemia	+	66
GP	Glutathione peroxidase	human transgene	ND	ND	67
nNOS	Neuronal nitric oxide synthase	homozygous (−/−) knockout	permanent focal cerebral ischemia	+	68
eNOS	Endothelial nitric oxide synthase	homozygous (−/−) knockout	permanent focal cerebral ischemia	−	69, 70
iNOS	Cytokine-inducible nitric oxide synthase	homozygous (−/−) knockout	ND	ND	71
p53	p53 protein	homozygous (−/−) knockout	permanent focal cerebral ischemia	+	72
sod-1	CuZn-superoxide dismutase	homozygous (−/−) heterozygous (+/−)	transient focal cerebral ischemia	−	73
sod-2	Mn-superoxide dismutase	heterozygous (+/−)	transient focal cerebral ischemia	−	74

+ = Neuronal protection; NP = no protection; ND = not determined; − = exacerbates ischemic infarction.

Fig. 2. Reduction of infarct volume in SOD-1 transgenic (Tg) mice after transient focal cerebral ischemia. Upper panel, representative photographs of brain sections at 24 h after 1 h of MCA occlusion in nontransgenic (nTg) and SOD-1 Tg mice. Infarcted areas were seen in the lateral part of caudate putamen and the dorsolateral cortex in nTg mice, while infarcted areas were only seen in caudate putamen with a small area of cerebral cortex in SOD-1 Tg mice. Middle and lower panels indicate infarct size of nTg and SOD-1 Tg mice. Values are mean ± SD (N = 6) $*p<0.05$, $**p<0.01$ (Tg vs. nTg mice by Student's t test).

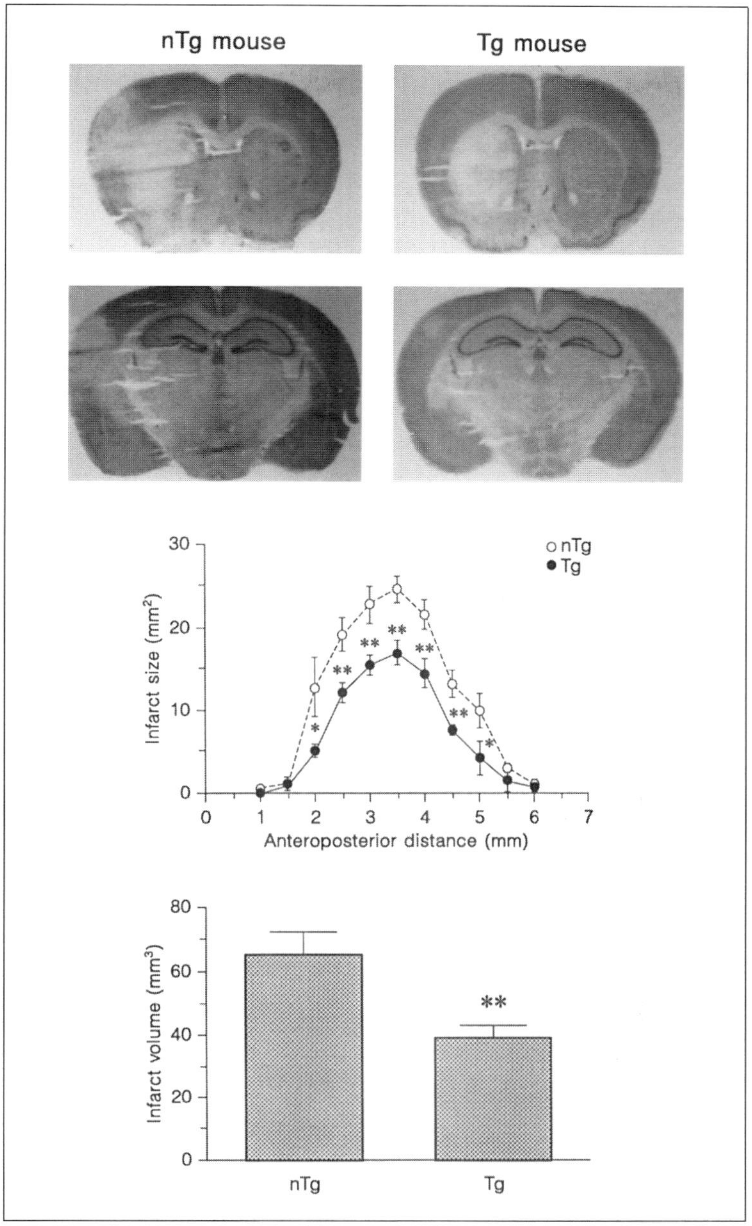
nTg mouse
Tg mouse
30
20
10
0
Infarct size (mm²)
○ nTg
● Tg
*
**
0 1 2 3 4 5 6 7
Anteroposterior distance (mm)
80
60
40
20
0
Infarct volume (mm³)
nTg
Tg

2

protects hippocampal CA_1 is unknown, it is possible that increased antioxidant enzyme activities in hippocampal neurons by bFGF overexpression [77] may account for the neuronal protection [78]. Tg mice in which neurons overexpress the human *BCL*-2 protein under the control of the neuron-specific enolase or phosphoglycerate kinase promotors, are protected against cerebral ischemia produced by permanent MCA occlusion [65]. *BCL*-2, a membranous protein that is encoded by *bcl-2*, a mammalian homologue of the nematode antiapoptotic gene ced-9 [79], has been known to interfere with neuronal apoptosis by acting as an antioxidant [80–82]. It has been demonstrated that the neurons that survive focal cerebral ischemic insult also express *BCL*-2 protein [83].

In a recent study, Lawrence et al. [84] have demonstrated that overexpression of *BCL*-2 with herpes simplex virus vectors protects the central nervous system neurons against focal cerebral ischemia in rats and glutamate-induced injury in hippocampal neurons in culture. Thus, these studies enforce the antioxidative concept in cerebral ischemia, since both Tg mice and rats overexpressing antioxidant protein *BCL*-2 are more resistant to cerebral ischemia-induced brain damage.

On the other hand, a limited number of mutant mice that contain a null mutation of a specific gene have been developed and used for the study of molecular and cellular mechanisms of cerebrovascular diseases. It has been demonstrated that ischemic infarction is significantly reduced in neuronal nitric oxide synthase (nNOS) knockout mice [68] that were developed by Huang et al. [85], clearly indicating that NO radicals produced by nNOS are major determinants of the pathogenesis of the infarct following permanent focal ischemia. These same investigators have recently developed knockout mice that are deficient in endothelial NOS [69, 70]. Although the inducible NOS (iNOS) has been implicated in cerebral ischemic damage [86] and the successful making of mutant mice deficient in iNOS [71], studies using these mice for cerebral ischemia are expected to be forthcoming. In another study using knockout mice, the ischemic infarct volume was significantly reduced in p53 mutant mice (both homozygous and heterozygous) following focal cerebral ischemia as compared to the wild-type [72]. Since the loss of p53 tumor suppressor gene has been shown to protect neurons from kainate-induced cell death [87], the neuronal protection offered by p53-deficient mutants may be related to the reduction of oxidative stress induced by kainate [88].

Using the knockout mutant mice, preliminary studies have been carried out to address the role of mouse cytosolic CuZn-SOD (*sod*-1) and Mn-SOD (*sod*-2) [73] in ischemic brain injury. It has recently been shown that ischemic infarct is significantly increased in mice that lack the *sod*-1 (homozygous and heterozygous) or *sod*-2 (heterozygous) gene [74, 89]. These studies, albeit preliminary, did point to the involvement of superoxide radicals in ischemic brain damage and to the important role these antioxidant enzymes play in neuronal protection following a focal ischemic insult.

Conclusion

It is now clear that oxidants play a major role in brain damage in cerebrovascular diseases. The successful making of *SOD*-1 Tg mice as well as *sod*-1, *sod*-2, nNOS knockout mutants, and many other Tg and knockout mutant mice has allowed stroke researchers and neuroscientists a unique opportunity to study the oxidative mechanisms underlying the complex neuronal responses to ischemic insults. It is clear that these genetically modified mice could also be useful for the study of neurodegenerative diseases and neurological disorders other than cerebrovascular diseases. Despite these successful beginnings, there are obvious advantages to using larger animal species (i.e., rats) for Tg animals and knockout mutants since many models for stroke and cerebrovascular disease have been mainly developed in rats [89]. The successful creation of Tg and knockout mutant rats will be an invaluable addition to the study of the mechanisms underlying ischemic brain damage in the well-established focal, thrombolytic and global ischemia models.

Acknowledgments

This work is supported by National Institutes of Health grants NS-14543, NS-25372, NS-36147, AG-08938, and NO1 NS-5-2334. I thank Ms. Cheryl Christensen for editorial assistance.

References

1 Kontos HA: Oxygen radicals in cerebral vascular injury. Circ Res 1985;57:508–516.

2 Hall ED, Braughler JM: Central nervous system trauma and stroke II. Physiological and pharmacological evidence for involvement of oxygen radicals and lipid peroxidation. Free Radic Biol Med 1989;6:303–313.

3 Siesjö BK, Agardh CD, Bengtsson F: Free radicals and brain damage. Cerebrovasc Brain Metab Rev 1989;1:165–211.

4 Chan PH: The role of oxygen radicals in brain injury and edema; in Chow CK (ed): Cellular Antioxidant Defense Mechanisms. Boca Raton, CRC Press, 1988, pp 89–109.

5 Chan PH: Antioxidant-dependent amelioration of brain injury: Role of CuZn-superoxide dismutase. J Neurotrauma 1992;9(suppl 2):417–432.

6 Chan PH, Chen S, Imaizumi S, Chu L, Kelleher JA, Gregory GA, Chan T: New insights into the role of oxygen radicals in cerebral ischemia; in Bazan NG, Braquet P, Ginsberg M (eds): Neurochemical Correlates of Cerebral Ischemia. Advances in Neurochemistry. New York, Plenum Press, 1992, vol 7, pp 277–294.

7 Boveris A, Chance B: The mitochondrial generation of hydrogen peroxide. Biochem J 1973;134: 707–716.

8 Meister A: Glutathione metabolism and its selective modification. J Biol Chem 1988;263:17205–17208.

9 Watson BD, Busto R, Goldberg WJ, Santison M, Yoshida S, Ginsberg MD: Lipid peroxidation in vivo induced by reversible global ischemia in rat brain. J Neurochem 1984;42:268–274.

10 Carney JM, Starke-Reed PE, Oliver CN, Landum RW, Cheng MS, Wu JF, Floyd RA: Reversal of age-related increase in brain protein oxidation decrease in enzyme activity, and loss in temporal and spatial memory by chronic administration of the spin-trapping compound N-tert-butyl-*L*-phenylnitrone. Proc Natl Acad Sci USA 1991;88:3633–3636.

11 Cathcart R, Schwiers E, Saul RL, Ames BN: Thymine glycol and thymidine glycol in human and rat urine: A possible assay for oxidative DNA damage. Proc Natl Acad Sci USA 1984;81:5633–5637.

12 Huang TT, Carlson EJ, Leadon SA, Epstein CJ: Relationship of resistance to oxygen free radicals to CuZn-superoxide dismutase activity in transgenic transfected and trisomic cells. FASEB J 1992; 6:903–910.

13 Oliver CN, Starke-Reed PE, Stadtman ER, Lui GJ, Carney JM, Floyd RA: Oxidative damage to brain proteins, loss of glutamine synthetase activity and production of free radicals during ischemia/reperfusion-induced injury to gerbil brain. Proc Natl Acad Sci USA 1990;87:5144–5147.

14 Malinski T, Bailey F, Zhang ZG, Chopp M: Nitric oxide measured by a porphyrinic microsensor in rat brain after transient middle cerebral artery occlusion. J Cereb Blood Flow Metab 1993;13: 355–358.

15 Tominaga T, Sato S, Ohnishi J, Ohnishi ST: Potentiation of nitric oxide formation following bilateral carotid occlusion and focal cerebral ischemia in the rat: In vivo detection of the nitric oxide radical by electron paramagnetic resonance spin trapping. Brain Res 1993;614:342–346.

16 Dugan LL, Sensi SL, Canzoniero LMT, Handran SD, Rothman SM, Lin T-S, Goldberg MP, Choi DW, Mitochondrial production of reactive oxygen species in cortical neurons following exposure to N-methyl-*D*-aspartate. J Neurosci 1995;15:6377–6388.

17 Lafon-Cazal M, Pietri S, Culcasi M, Bockaert J: NMDA-dependent superoxide production and neurotoxicity. Nature 1993;364:535–537.

18 Fabian RH, DeWitt DS, Kent TA: In vivo detection of superoxide anion production by the brain using a cytochrome c electrode. J Cereb Blood Flow Metab 1995;15:242–247.

19 Bindokas VP, Jordán J, Lee CC, Miller RJ: Superoxide produduction in rat hippocampal neurons: Selective imaging with hydroethidine. J Neurosci 1996;16:1324–1336.

20 Patel M, Day BJ, Crapo JD, Fridovich I, McNamara JO: Requirement for superoxide in excitotoxic cell death. Neuron 1996;16:345–355.

21 Dawson TM, Dawson VL, Snyder SH: A novel neuronal messenger molecule in brain: The free radical, nitric oxide. Ann Neurol 1992;32:297–311.

22 Murphy S, Simmons ML, Agullo L, Garcia A, Feinstein DL, Galea E, Reis DJ, MincGolomb D, Schwartz JP: Synthesis of nitric oxide in CNS glial cells. Trends Neurosci 1993;16:323–328.

23 Beckman JS, Beckman TW, Chen J, Marshall PA, Freeman BA: Apparent hydroxyl radical production by peroxynitrite: Implications for endothelial injury from nitric oxide and superoxide. Proc Natl Acad Sci USA 1990;87:1620–1624.

24 Hue RT, Padmaja S: The reaction of NO with superoxide. Free Radic Res Comun 1993;18:195–199.

25 Beckman JS, Carson M, Smith CD, Koppenol WH: ALS, SOD and peroxynitrite (letter).Nature 1993;364:584.

26 Tanaka K, Fukuuchi Y, Gomi S, Mihara B, Shirai T, Nogawa S, Nozaki H, Nagata E: Inhibition of nitric oxide synthesis impairs autoregulation of local cerebral blood flow in the rat. Neuroreport 1993;4:267–270.

27 Prado R, Watson BD: Effects of nitric oxide synthase inhibition on cerebral blood flow following bilateral carotid artery occlusion and recirculation in the rat. J Cereb Blood Flow Metab 1993;13: 720–723.

28 Zhang F, Iadecola C: Nitroprusside improves blood flow and reduces brain damage after focal ischemia. Neuroreport 1993;4:559–562.

29 Iadecola C: Regulation of the cerebral microcirculation during neural activity: Is nitric oxide the missing link? Trends Neurosci 1993;16:206–214.

30 Wei EP, Moskowitz MA, Boccalini P, Kontos HA: Calcitonin gene-related peptide mediates nitroglycerin and sodium nitroprusside-induced vasodilation in feline cerebral arterioles. Circ Res 1992;70:1313–1319.

31 Pelligrino DA, Koenig HM, Albrecht RF: Nitric oxide synthesis and regional cerebral blood flow responses to hypercapnia and hypoxia in the rat. J Cereb Blood Flow Metab 1993;13:80–87.

32 Dawson VL, Dawson TM, Bartely DA, Uhl GR, Snyder SH: Mechanisms of nitric oxide-mediated neurotoxicity in primary brain cultures. J Neurosci 1993;13:2651–2661.

33 Nagafuji T, Matsui T, Koide T, Asano T: Blockade of nitric oxide formation by N^{w}-nitro-*L*-arginine mitigates ischemic brain edema and susequent cerebral infarction in rats. Neurosci Lett 1992;147:159–162.

34 Kiedrowski L, Costa E, Wroblewski JT: Glutamate recetor agonists stimulate nitric oxide synthase in primary cultures of cerebellar granule cells. J Neurochem 1991;58:335–341.

35 Lei SZ, Pan ZH, Aggarwal SK, Chen HSV, Lipton SA: Effect of nitric oxide production on the redox modulatory site of the NMDA receptor-channel complex. Neuron 1992;8:1087–1099.

36 Lipton SA, Choi YB, Pan ZH, Lei SZ, Chen HS, Sucher NJ, Loscalzo J, Singel DJ, Stamler JS: A redox-based mechanism for the neuroprotective and neurodestructive effects of nitric oxide and related nitroso-compounds. Nature 1993;364:626–632.

37 Troy CM, Derossi D, Prochiantz A, Greene LA, Shelanski ML: Downregulation of Cu/Zn superoxide dismutase leads to cell death via the nitric oxide-peroxynitrite pathway. J Neurosci 1996;16:253–261.

38 Oberley LW: Superoxide Dismutase. Boca Raton, CRC Press, 1982, vol 1, pp 1–141.

39 Lieman-Hurwitz J, Dafni N, Lavie V, Groner Y: Human cytoplasmic superoxide dismutase cDNA clone: A probe for studying the molecular biology of Down syndrome. Proc Natl Acad Sci USA 1982;79:2808–2811.

40 Levanon D, Lieman-Hurwitz J, Dafni N, Wigderson M, Sherman L, Bernstein Y, Laver-Rudich Z, Danciger E, Stein O, Groner Y: Architecture and anatomy of the chromosomal locus in human chromosome 21 encoding in the Cu/Zn superoxide dismutase. EMBO J 1985;4:77–84.

41 Marklund SL: Human copper-containing superoxide dismutase of high molecular weight. Proc Natl Acad Sci USA 1982;79:7634–7638.

42 Cerchiari EL, Hoel TM, Safar P, Sclabassi RJ: Protective effects of combined superoxide dismutase and deferoxamine on recovery of cerebral blood flow and function after cardiac arrest in dogs. Stroke 1987;18:869–878.

43 Forsman M, Fleischer JE, Midle JH, Stten PA, Michenfelder JD: Superoxide dismutase and catalase failed to improve neurologic outcome after complete cerebral ischemia in the dog. Acta Anaesthesiol Scand 1988;32:152–155.

44 Pigott JP, Donovan DL, Fink JA, Sharp WV: Experimental pharmacologic cerebroprotection. J Vasc Surg 1988;7:625–630.

45 Lui TH, Beckman JS, Freeman BA, Hogan EL, Hsu CY: Polyethylene glycol-conjugated superoxide dismutase and catalase reduce ischemic brain injury. Am J Physiol 1989;256:H589–H593.

46 Uyama O, Shiratsuki N, Matsuyama T, Nakanishi T, Mutsumoto Y, Yamada T, Narita M, Sugita M: Protective effects of superoxide dismutase on acute reperfusion injury of gerbil brain. Free Radic Biol Med 1990;8:265–268.

47 Imaizumi S, Woolworth V, Fishman RA, Chan PH: Liposome-entrapped superoxide dismutase reduces cerebral infarction in cerebral ischemia in rats. Stroke 1990;21:1312–1317.

48 Schurer L, Grogaard B, Gerdin B, Arfors KE: Superoxide dismutase does not prevent delayed hypoperfusion after incomplete cerebral ischemia in the rat. Acta Neurochir 1990;103:163–170.

49 Kitagawa K, Matsumoto M, Oda T, Niinobe M, Hata R, Handa N, Fukunaga R, Isaka Y, Kimura K, Maeda H: Free radical generation during brief periods of cerebral ischemia may trigger delayed neuronal death. Neuroscience 1990;35:551–558.

50 Haun SE, Kirsch JR, Helfaer MA, Kubos KL, Traystman RJ: Polyethylene glycol-conjugated superoxide dismutase fails to augment brain superoxide dismutase activity in piglets. Stroke 1991;22:655–659.

51 Phelan AM, Lange DG: Ischemia/reperfusion-induced changes in membrane fluidity characteristics of brain capillary endothelial cells and its prevention by liposomal -incorporated superoxide dismutase. Biochim Biophys Acta 1991;1067:97–102.
52 Armstead WM, Mirro R, Thelin OP, Shibata M, Zuckerman SL, Shanklin DR, Busija DW, Leffler CW: Polyethylene glycol superoxide dismutase and catalase attenuate increased blood-brain barrier permeability after ischemia in piglets. Stroke 1992;23:755–762.
53 Ohtsuki T, Matsumoto M, Kuwabara K, Kitagawa K, Suzuki K, Taniguchi N, Kamada T: Influence of oxidative stress on induced tolerance to ischemia in gerbil hippocampal neurons. Brain Res 1992; 599:246–252.
54 Tasdemiroglu E, Chistenberry PD, Ardell JL, Chronister RB, Taylor AE: Effect of superoxide dismutase on acute reperfusion injury of the rabbit brain. Acta Neurochir 1993;120:180–186.
55 Takeda Y, Hashimoto H, Kosaka F, Hirakawa M, Inoue M: Albimin-binding superoxide dismutase with a prolonged half-life reduces reperfusion brain injury. Am J Physiol 1993;264:H1708–H1715.
56 Leblanc MH, Vig V, Randhawa T, Smith EE, Parker CC, Brown EG: Use of polyethylene glycol-bound superoxide dismutase, polyethylene glycol-bound catalase, and nimodipine to prevent hypoxic ischemic injury to the brain of newborn pigs. Crit Care Med 1993;21:252–259.
57 He YY, Hsu CY, Ezrin AM, Miller MS: Polyethylene glycol-conjugated superoxide dismutase in focal cerebral ischemia-reperfusion. Am J Physiol 1993;265:H252–H256.
58 Chan PH, Epstein CJ, Kinouchi H, Imaizumi S, Carlson E, Chen SF: Role of superoxide dismutase in ischemic brain injury: Reduction of edema and infarction in transgenic mice following focal cerebral ischemia. Prog Brain Res 1993;96:97–104.
59 Chan PH, Longar S, Fishman RA: Protective effects of liposome-entrapped superoxide dismutase on post-traumatic brain edema. Ann Neurol 1987;21:540–547.
60 Gordon JW, Scangos GA, Plotkin DJ, Barbosa JA, Ruddle FH: Genetic transformation of mouse embryos by microinjection of purified DNA. Proc Natl Acad Sci USA 1980;77:12:7380–7384.
61 Thomas KR, Capecchi MR: Site-directed mutagenesis by gene targeting in mouse embryo-derived stem cells. Cell 1987;51:503–512.
62 Kinouchi H, Mizui T, Carlson EJ, Epstein CJ, Chan PH: Alteration of cerebral infarction and antioxidant levels in focal cerebral ischemia in transgenic mice overexpressing CuZn-SOD. The First International Neurotrauma Symposium, Fukushima, May 14–17, 1991.
63 Yang G, Chan PH, Chen J, Carlson E, Chen SF, Weinstein P, Epstein CJ, Kamii H: Human copper-zinc superoxide dismutase transgenic mice are highly resistant to reperfusion injury after focal cerebral ischemia. Stroke 1994;25:165–170.
64 Chan PH, Kamii H, Yang G, Garni J, Epstein CJ, Carslon E, Reola L: Brain infraction is not reduced in SOD–1 transgenic mice after a permanent focal cerebral ischemia. Neuroreport 1993; 5:293–296.
65 Martinou JC, Dubois-Dauphin M, Staple JK, Rodriguez I, Frankowski H, Missotten M, Albertini P, Talabot D, Catsicas S, Pietra C: Overexpression of BCL-2 in transgenic mice protects neurons from naturally occurring cell death and experimental ischemia. Neuron 1994;13:1017–1030.
66 MacMillan V, Judge D, Wiseman A, Settle D, Swain J, Davis J: Mice expressing a bovine basic fibroblast growth factor transgene in the brain show increased resistance to hypoxemic-ischemic cerebral damage. Stroke 1993;24:1735–1739.
67 Mitochnitchenko O, Palnitkar U, Philbert M, Inouye M: Thermosensitive phenotype of transgenic mice overproducing human glutathione peroxidases. Proc Natl Acad Sci USA 1995;92:8120–8124.
68 Huang Z, Huang PL, Panahian N, Dalkara T, Fishman M, Moskowitz MA: Effects of cerebral ischemia in mice deficient in neuronal nitric oxide synthase. Science 1994;265:1883–1885.
69 Huang PL, Huang Z, Mashimo H, Bloch KD, Moskowitz MA, Bevan JA, Fishman MC: Hypertension in mice lacking the gene for endothelial nitric oxide synthase. Nature 1995;377:239–242.
70 Huang Z, Huang PL, Fishman MC, Moskowitz MA: Focal cerebral ischemia in mice deficient in either endothelial (eNOS) or neuronal nitric oxide (nNOS) synthase (abstract). Stroke 1996;27:173.
71 MacMicking JD, Nathan C, Hom G, Chartrain N, Fletcher DS, Trumbauer M, Stevens K, Xie Q-W, Sokol K, Hutchinson N, Chen H, Mudgett JS: Altered responses to bacterial infection and endotoxic shock in mice lacking inducible nitric oxide synthase. Cell 1995;81:641–650.

72 Crumrine RC, Thomas AL, Morgan PF: Attenuation of p53 expression protects against focal ischemic damage in transgenic mice. J Cereb Blood Flow Metab 1994;14:887–891.
73 Kondo T, Reaume A, Huang TT, Carlson E, Chen S, Scott R, Epstein CJ, Chan PH: Target disruption of CuZn-superoxide dismutase gene in mice causes exacerbation of cerebral infraction and neurological deficits after focal cerebral ischemia and reperfusion. Soc Neurosci Abstr 1995; 21:1268.
74 Mikawa S, Li Y, Huang TT, Carlson E, Chen S, Kondo T, Murakami K, Epstein CJ, Chan PH: Cerebral infarction is exacerbated in mitochondrial maganese superoxide dismutase (Sod-2) knockout mutant mice after focal cerebral ischemia and reperfusion. Soc Neurosci Abstr 1995;21: 1268.
75 Kinouchi H, Epstein CJ, Mizui T, Carlson EJ, Chen SF, Chan PH: Attenuation of focal cerebral ischemic injury in transgenic mice overexpressing CuZn superoxide dismutase. Proc Natl Acad Sci USA 1991;88:11158–11162.
76 Kamii H, Kinouchi H, Chen SF, Sharp FR, Epstein CJ, Chan PH: SOD-1 transgenic mice: An application to the study of ischemic brain injury; in Ohnishi ST (ed): Membrane-Linked Diseases. Boca Raton, CRC Press, 1995, vol 4, pp 423–431.
77 Mattson MP, Lovell MA, Furukawa K, Markesbery WR: Neurotrophic factors attenuate glutamate-induced accumulation of peroxides, elevation of intracellular Ca^{2+} concentration, and neurotoxicity and increase antioxidant enzyme activities in hippocampal neurons. J Neurochem 1995;65:1740–1751.
78 Freese A, Findlestein SP, DiFiglia M: Basic fibroblast growth factor protects striatal neurons in vitro from NMDA-receptor mediated excitotoxicity. Brain Res 1992;575:351–355.
79 Yuan J, Shaham S, Ledoux S, Ellis HM, Horvitz HR: The *C. elegans* cell death gene ced-3 encodes a protein similar to mammalian interleukin-1-beta-converting enzyme. Cell 1993;75:641–652.
80 Kane DJ, Sarafian TA, Anton R, Hahn H, Gralla EB, Valentine JS, Ord T, Bredesen D: Bcl-2 inhibition of neural death: Decreased generation of reactive oxygen species. Science 1993;262: 1274–1277.
81 Greenlund LJ, Korsmeyer SJ, Johnson EM Jr: Role of BCL-2 in the survival and function of developing and mature sympathetic neurons. Neuron 1995;15:649–661.
82 Zhong LT, Sarafian T, Kane DJ, Charles AC, Mah SP, Edwards RH, Bredesen DE: bcl-2 inhibits death of central neural cells induced by multiple agents. Proc Natl Acad Sci USA 1993;90:4533–4537.
83 Chen J, Graham SH, Chan PH, Lan J, Shou RL, Simon RP: bcl-2 is expressed in neurons that survive focal ischemia in the rat. Neuroreport 1995;6:394–398.
84 Lawrence MS, Ho DY, Sun GH, Steinberg GK, Sapolsky RM: Overexpression of Bcl-2 with herpes simplex virus vectors protects CNS neurons against neurological insults in vitro and in vivo. J Neurosci 1996;16:486–496.
85 Huang PL, Dawson PM, Bredt DS, Snyder SH, Fishman ME: Targeted disruption of the neuronal nitric oxide synthase gene. Cell 1993;75:1273–1286.
86 Iadecola C, Xu X, Zhang F, El-Fakahany EE, Ross ME: Marked induction of calcium-independent nitric oxide synthase activity after focal cerebral ischemia. J Cereb Blood Flow Metab 1995;15: 52–59.
87 Morrison RS, Wenzel HJ, Kinoshita Y, Robbins CA, Donehower LA, Schwartzkroin PA: Loss of the p53 tumor suppressor gene protects neurons from kainate-induced cell death. J Neurosci 1996; 16:1337–1345.
88 Li Y, Huang T-T, Carlson EJ, Melov S, Ursell PC, Olson JL, Noble LJ, Yoshimura MP, Berger C, Chan PH, Wallace DC, Epstein CJ: Dilated cardiomyopathy and neonatal lethality in mutant mice lacking manganese superoxide dismutase. Nat Genet 1995;11:376–381.
89 Ginsberg MD: Models of cerebral ischemia in the rodent; in Schurr A, Rigor BM (eds): Cerebral Ischemia and Resuscitation. Boca Raton, CRC Press, 1990, pp 1–15.

Pak H. Chan, PhD, Department of Neurological Surgery, University of California,
521 Parnassus, C-224, San Francisco, CA 94143-0651 (USA)

Hsu CY (ed): Ischemic Stroke: From Basic Mechanisms to New Drug Development.
Monogr Clin Neurosci. Basel, Karger, 1998, vol 16, pp 28–45

Nitric Oxide in Cerebrovascular Regulation and Ischemia

Turgay Dalkara, Michael A. Moskowitz

Stroke and Neurovascular Regulation Laboratory, Department of Neurology and Neurosurgical Service, Massachusetts General Hospital, Harvard Medical School, Charlestown, Mass., USA

Nitric oxide (NO) was first recognized as an inorganic air pollutant present in exhaust gas and cigarette smoke. It was a surprise for scientists to discover that this pollutant was in fact a biologically relevant molecule that mediated the bactericidal action of macrophages [1, 2]. NO was also identified as a mediator of vasodilation, operating as a signaling molecule rather than through a cytotoxic mode of action [3, 4]. It is now accepted that NO or a related nitroso compound is the endothelium-derived relaxing factor (EDRF) and NO is one of the major molecules regulating vascular tone and blood pressure [5]. Following these discoveries, NO was shown to be a ubiquitous molecule in mammalian tissues and plays a role in a broad spectrum of physiological functions [6]. NO has emerged as the first example of a new class of inorganic gaseous neuromediators in part related to the finding that most of the regulatory actions of NO are mediated via activation of guanylate cyclase and that high cyclic GMP levels are found in the cerebellum [7, 8].

Under most conditions, small puffs of NO generated by calcium-dependent activation of constitutive NO synthase (NOS) mediate the physiological functions of NO [6, 9]. Following its generation by NOS, NO readily diffuses beyond its site of origin to influence adjacent cells. Due to its high affinity for iron and thiol groups, NO binds to several target molecules and modifies cellular processes [8, 10]. When continuously synthesized in great abundance however, NO can be cytotoxic [10, 11]. Sustained NO production is achieved by calcium-independent inducible isoform of NOS (iNOS) in activated macrophages and other inflammatory cells [1, 12]. In addition to its bactericidal and tumoricidal actions, NO generated by iNOS may play a cytotoxic role in diseases such as multiple sclerosis [13]. However, under energy-compromised conditions, neuronal NOS (nNOS) can also provide a sustained NO generation and participate in neuronal death [10, 14–16]. According to this hypothesis, an unregulated rise in intracellular calcium augments neuronal NO synthesis by constitutive NOS leading to a build up in NO concentrations to toxic levels. Since intracellular calcium levels rapidly increase during cerebral ischemia, this hypothesis predicts that a sustained NO generation in neurons can participate in ischemic neuronal death. Accordingly, NOS inhibitors were tried in various ischemia models with the hope of reducing ischemic damage; but conflicting results were reported [see 17 for review]. We proposed that NO's role was complex in ischemia because it dilated cerebral blood vessels and increased blood flow to ischemic tissue in addition to its cytotoxic action [17]. Consequently, inhibition of both endothelial and neuronal NOS probably causes opposing actions and the net effect of non-selective NOS inhibitors on stroke outcome is unpredictable and depends upon the protocol used.

Recently, development of mutant mice with deletions of the gene encoding nNOS or endothelial NOS (eNOS) provided an opportunity to dissect the complex role of NO in cerebral ischemia. The data from these studies strongly suggest that NO produced by neurons contributes to ischemic damage whereas NO generated by the endothelium affects stroke outcome more favorably [18, 19]. The evidence will be reviewed below.

Synthesis and Metabolism of NO

NO is synthesized from the guanidino nitrogen of *L*-arginine and molecular oxygen by NO synthase [see 20 for review]. At least three isoforms of the NOS enzyme have been identified: neuronal (type 1) and endothelial (type 3), which are constitutive, and an inducible isoform (type 2) originally isolated from murine macrophages [21–23]. The inducible NOS characterized in human hepatocytes and articular chondrocytes may represent a distinct isoform [24, 25]. All isoforms possess both a reductase and oxygenase domain separated by a calmodulin-binding region. The reaction requires NADPH and produces stoichiometric amounts of citrulline and NO following a five electron-oxidation of *L*-arginine. The oxidation takes place in a dimeric protein with two identical subunits containing two flavins, tetrahydrobiopterin and a heme complex [20]. The amino acid sequence of the reductase domain is closely homologous to cytochrome P_{450} reductase, which suggests a similar electron flow for both enzymes [26]. All three isoforms possess NADPH-diaphorase activity, the presence of which has been used to infer the localization of NOS [27]. Recently, it was reported that NADPH-diaphorase activity disclosed eNOS-containing cells after gluteraldehyde rather than formaldehyde fixation [28].

The constitutive isoforms are calcium/calmodulin-dependent and activated by intracellular calcium transients. An increase in intracellular calcium concentration from 100 to 500 nM changes the rate of NO synthesis from <5 to $>95\%$ of maximum [29]. This Ca^{2+} sensitivity is typical for a calmodulin-activated enzyme. On the other hand, calmodulin is very tightly bound to the inducible isoform, making it insensitive to fluctuations in cytoplasmic calcium levels [30]. Normally, NOS activity in macrophages is undetectable and stimulation of iNOS gene transcription by endotoxins and cytokines is required. Once expressed, iNOS is continuously active and leads to a long-lasting (several hours to day) NO generation compared to calcium-dependent NO synthesis lasting a few minutes [12].

Under normal conditions, only constitutive NOS can be detected in brain using immunohistochemical methods. nNOS is detected in neurons and perivascular nerves, and eNOS in cerebrovascular endothelium and in a small population of neurons [28, 31, 32]. Very low levels of nNOS are detected in astrocytes [33]. However, astrocytes, microglia, vascular smooth muscle and endothelial cells can express iNOS upon induction [33–37]. The genes encoding the endothelial, neuronal and inducible proteins have been cloned and sequenced. The eNOS gene was assigned to chromosome 7 whereas the neuronal and inducible genes were located on chromosomes 12 and 17, respectively [38–40].

Once formed, NO readily diffuses out of cells. Rapid removal by metalloproteins like hemoglobin limits its spread to a few hundred microns and shortens its half-life to the order of seconds [9, 41]. Absence of hemoglobin prolongs NO's half-life and increases its tissue levels. Formation of S-nitrosothiol adducts may stabilize the labile NO radical and prolong its biological half-life. Sulfhydryl groups in proteins (e.g., albumin) represent a rich source of reduced thiol, and S-nitroso-proteins form readily under physiological conditions [42]. NO converts hemoglobin to methemoglobin in red cells, which is instantly reduced back to hemoglobin and nitrate. Accordingly, urinary nitrate and nitrite levels can be useful as an indirect measure of NO metabolism [43]. Under physiological conditions, rapid degradation of superoxide by superoxide dismutase renders the interaction of NO with superoxide less likely [44]. The rate constants for the formation of peroxynitrite anions is three times faster than for the SOD reaction (6.7×10^9 vs. 2×10^9 m^{-1} s^{-1}) and therefore, favors peroxynitrate formation. Available data suggest that tissue NO levels are essentially controlled by mechanisms regulating NO biosynthesis [20]. In vitro experiments imply that NO inhibits NOS activity by interacting with NOS or its cofactors [45]. However, whether this inhibitory feedback mechanism occurs in vivo is not known.

Molecular Mechanisms of NO Action

Interactions with Heme Groups

Cyclic GMP formation may mediate the actions of NO via activation of the heme-containing enzyme guanylate cyclase, following formation of an NO-heme complex [6, 20]. However, cGMP-dependent mechanisms may be operational primarily in cells adjacent to those generating NO because intracellular calcium levels sufficient to activate NO synthase inhibit guanylate cyclase [29, 46]. Blood vessels may provide such an example. Vasodilatory neuromediators like acetylcholine or bradykinin raise intracellular calcium and stimulate endothelial NOS activity to release NO or a related nitrosothiol (EDRF) from endothelial cells. NO, in turn, enhances cGMP synthesis in smooth muscle cells which initiates a cascade that relaxes vascular smooth muscle [9, 47]. Nitrovasodilators such as nitroglycerin, nitroprusside or SIN-1 raise cGMP in vascular smooth muscle by directly liberating or donating NO [48]. Platelet inhibition, neurotransmission and penile erection are also mediated by cGMP-dependent mechanisms [6, 10]. cGMP levels are elevated during neuronal activity in various parts of the brain including cerebellum, cerebral cortex and hippocampus [41]. However, the role of cGMP here is unclear. Formation of NO-heme complexes in cyclooxygenase may increase enzyme activity and stimulate prostaglandin production as well [49].

Interactions with Thiol Groups

NO may also react reversibly with thiol groups to modulate the activity of certain proteins [42]. Some antimicrobial effects of NO, inhibition of N-methyl-*D*-aspartate (NMDA) receptor activity, regulation of ADP-ribosylation and inhibition of glyceraldehyde-3-phosphate dehydrogenase are examples of the latter mechanism [50]. NO can be interconverted among three redox forms [nitrosonium (NO^+), nitric oxide ($NO^{\bullet}$) and nitroxyl anion (NO^-)] under physiological conditions [51]. These redox forms favor different effector interactions. For example, $NO^{\bullet}$ is required for activation of guanylate cyclase and also may be neurotoxic whereas NO^+ down regulates NMDA receptor activity, thereby affording neuroprotection [51]. NO donors may also exert opposing actions depending upon the redox form of released NO. For example, Lipton et al. [52] proposed that sodium nitroprusside protected neurons because it generates NO^+ but can be converted to the $NO^{\bullet}$ toxic pathway after reduction with cysteine. Tissue redox state and pH favors different redox forms of NO and consequently different target molecules may be activated within cellular compartments and under various pathological conditions. The hypotheses remain uncertain at the present time because of difficulties in detection of NO and its redox forms in vivo currently. It also remains possible that some of these reactions may provide important signaling mechanisms essential for physiological cell regulation.

NOS Inhibition

Most researchers use NOS inhibitors to investigate the role of NO in various physiological and pathological conditions. The most widely studied inhibitors are the substrate analogs of *L*-arginine such as nitro-*L*-arginine methyl ester (*L*-NAME), nitro-*L*-arginine (*L*-NA) and monomethyl-*L*-arginine (*L*-NMMA). In most instances, the conversion of *L*-arginine and molecular oxygen to citrulline and NO is blocked competitively, although noncompetitive inhibition may occur depending upon dosage and treatment duration [53–55]. Like NOS activity itself, enzyme inhibition is enantiomerically specific.

L-NAME, *L*-NA and *L*-NMMA inhibit both the constitutively expressed and inducible enzymes and do not discriminate between the neuronal and endothelial isoforms [56]. It is notable however that *L*-NA displays a marked preference for the constitutively expressed protein whereas *L*-NMMA is reportedly more potent and effective against the inducible protein [57]. Recently, 7-nitroindazole was reported to inhibit neuronal NOS potently without increasing blood pressure [58] or blocking acetylcholine relaxation of pial vessels [59], suggesting that it may selectively inhibit the neuronal form in vivo; however, it has a similar IC_{50} for nNOS (0.9 μM) and eNOS (0.7 μM) in vitro [60]. A number of new inhibitors reported to be selective have been introduced recently [61, 62]. Aminoguanidine has drawn particular attention as a selective iNOS inhibitor, considering the putative role of iNOS in many diseases [63]. However, the molecular basis of its selectivity is not clear and it has actions on several other enzymes too.

NOS inhibitors exhibit other effects such as muscarinic antagonist action [64], cytochrome c reduction [65] and blockade of endothelium-independent vasodilation. In addition, *L*-NMMA competes with *L*-arginine uptake [66], can be metabolized by endothelial cells to *L*-citrulline which in turn serves as a precursor for NO synthesis by conversion to *L*-arginine [67]. Inhibition of NOS activity by inhibiting flavoproteins, calmodulin and synthesis of tetrahydrobiopterin is also possible but these agents may exert nonspecific effects [68].

Functions of NO in the Brain

Regulation of Neuronal Activity

Elevations in NO and cGMP levels occur during neuronal activity in various parts of the brain including cerebellum, cerebral cortex and hippocampus [41]. Glutamate-induced intracellular calcium increase, mostly through NMDA receptors, may account for the observed increase in NO and subsequent enhancement of cGMP levels in neighboring cells and in the presynaptic terminal from which glutamate is released [7, 69]. Recent evidence indicates that cGMP may lead to direct gating of channels and it may also modulate several cellular functions through activation of cGMP-dependent protein kinases and modulation of phosphodiesterases [41]. There is also evidence suggesting a role for NO-induced cGMP augmentation in synaptic plasticity (e.g. long-term potentiation) [70, 71]. Failure of NO donors or NOS inhibitors to cause obvious changes in membrane potential and neuronal firing initially led to the idea that NO did not have an effect on electrophysiological behavior of neurons. However, increasing evidence indicates that NO may modulate firing of several neuronal groups such as corticothalamic oscillatory neurons [72] and may act on ion channels (e.g. calcium currents), neurotransmitter release and uptake [73, 74]. Several reports suggest that NO has neuroendocrine functions [e.g. 75].

Regulation of Cerebral Blood Flow

Topical or systemic administration of NOS inhibitors constricts cerebral arteries and reduces rCBF, suggesting that NO contributes to normal vascular tonus [76–79]. In parallel with this, intravenous infusion of *L*-arginine, like NO, leads to pial vessel dilation and blood flow increases within normal rat brain [80, 81]. NO's contribution to basal tone varies among brain regions and species. Available evidence suggests that both neuronal and endothelial NO participate [82].

NO has also been proposed as one of the mediators of the blood flow augmentation during moderate hypercapnia and of metabolism-flow coupling [83, 84]. In both cases, neuronally-generated NO rather than the NO of endothelial origin has been shown to contribute to vasodilation [85–87]. NO may also participate in rCBF enhancement induced by NMDA applications [88] and cortical spreading depression [89].

NO-Mediated Neurotoxicity

NOS-containing neurons are resistant to NMDA toxicity as well as to destruction in Huntington's disease and ischemia [90, 91]. These neurons comprise only 1–2% of all the neurons in the cerebral cortex, corpus striatum and hippocampus; however, they extensively branch and are thought to kill neighboring neurons when they produce NO in excessive amounts [16, 27, 92]. NO may cause cytotoxicity by disrupting mitochondrial respiration due to inhibition of aconitase and complex I and II of mitochondrial electron transport [see 10, 11] (fig. 1). NO acts on these enzymes through formation of iron-NO complexes. The inhibition of glyceraldehyde-3-phosphate dehydrogenase by NO may also have detrimental consequences by depressing glycolysis and reducing intracellular glutathione levels [50].

In addition to disrupting cellular metabolism, NO inhibits DNA synthesis by depressing ribonucleotide reductase activity [93]. NO also damages DNA structure by several possible ways including DNA nitration, deamination and oxidation [94]. Recently, it has been proposed that DNA damage plays a central role in NO toxicity [95]. According to this hypothesis, DNA damage activates normal reparative mechanisms such as poly-ADP ribose synthase, which can deplete the cell of (already reduced) ATP and nicotinamide dinucleotide, hence further compromising cellular energy metabolism. Other than through promoting necrotic cell death, NO may be one of the mediators inducing programmed cell death. NO donors and possibly endogenously produced NO have been shown to cause apoptosis in chondrocytes [96], mastocytomas [97] and macrophages [98]. Apoptotic cell death was demonstrated in global [99, 100] and transient focal ischemia [101–103]. Whether or not NO triggers neuronal apoptosis in ischemia is currently unknown.

Available evidence also indicates that formation of peroxynitrite ($ONOO^-$) by interaction of NO with superoxide anion may be a major pathway through which NO mediates cell death [104, 105]. NO may outcompete superoxide dismutase to interact with superoxide when produced in excessive amounts under pathological conditions [106]. $ONOO^-$ anion also decomposes to other reactive oxygen species, hydroxyl radical-like product and nitrogen dioxide, which is a potent activator of lipid peroxidation. Peroxynitrite anion also facilitates S-nitrosylation of proteins. Especially in a superoxide-rich environment, NO may release intracellular iron thereby triggering the Haber-Weiss reaction and formation of reactive oxygen species [11]. NOS produces reactive oxygen species instead of NO when tissue *L*-arginine is depleted [107]. However, there is evidence that NO may be a neuroprotective agent by scavenging superoxide and iron and hence decreasing superoxide toxicity [108, 109].

In summary, NO may be cytotoxic by directly inhibiting enzymes that catalyze vital cellular functions such as energy metabolism and DNA synthesis through its well-known affinity for iron and thiol groups, or indirectly by $ONOO^-$ formation or iron release. It is likely that different cytotoxic mecha-

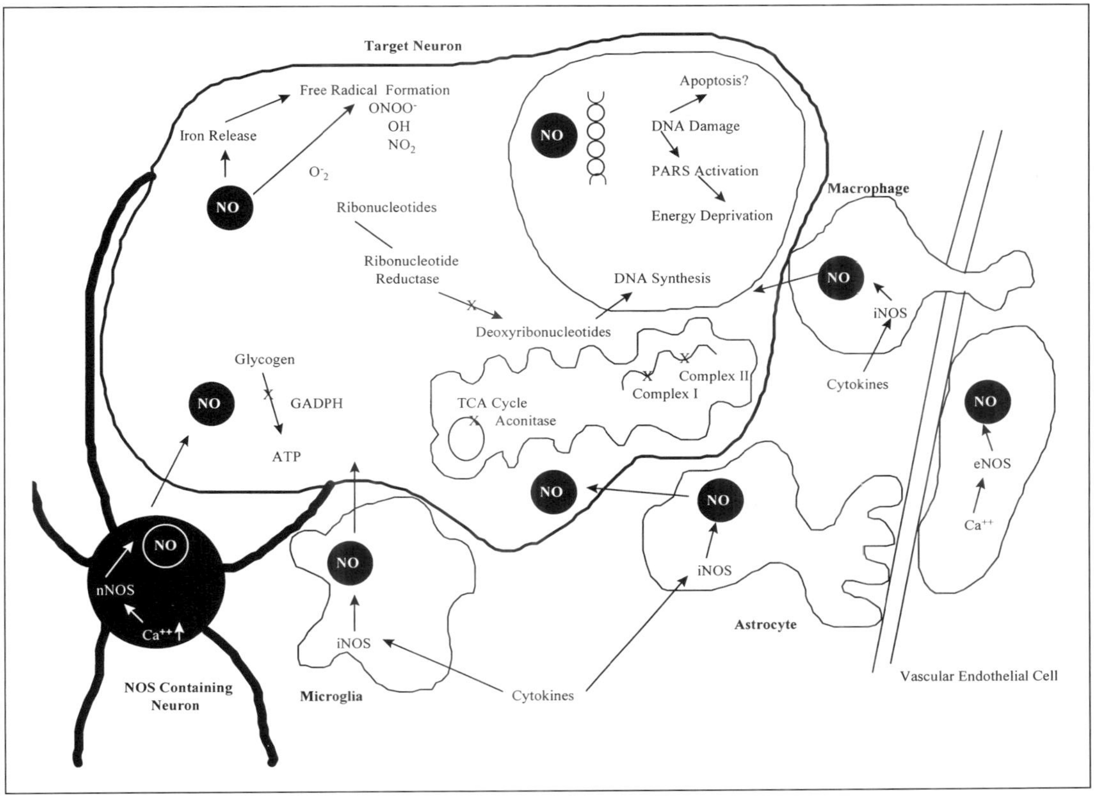

Fig. 1. NO-mediated neurotoxicity: NO is generated in vascular endothelium and NOS-containing neurons at the onset of ischemia due to a rise in intracellular calcium. Vascular NO may improve ischemic blood flow and be neuroprotective but sustained synthesis of NO in neurons and NO generated in microglia, astrocytes and invading macrophages after induction of iNOS is cytotoxic. NO causes cell death by inhibiting mitochondrial respiration (complex I and II, aconitase), glycolysis (glyceraldehyde-3-phosphate dehydrogenase (GAPHD)) and DNA synthesis (ribonucleotide reductase). NO leads to DNA damage which may end up in energy depletion due to activation of poly(ADP-ribose) synthase (PARS) or in apoptosis. NO may also cause free radical damage by formation of peroxynitrite, hydroxyl radical, nitrogen dioxide and by iron catalyzed Haber-Weiss reaction. Figure produced by Dr. H. Bolay.

nisms may prevail under different pathological conditions. For example, depending on the availability of O_2 and generation of superoxide, the mechanisms mediating NO toxicity may differ between permanent and transient focal and also between the early and late phases of ischemia particularly when NO is generated by constitutive NOS and not by iNOS activity.

NO and the NMDA Receptor

NO was proposed as the neurotoxic agent mediating NMDA toxicity [15]. Studies in dissociated cell cultures showed that NOS inhibitors effectively blocked NMDA-induced cell death whereas *L*-arginine depletion attenuated NMDA receptor-mediated toxicity [15]. NMDA toxicity was also blocked by reducing NOS catalytic activity by calmodulin antagonists, flavoprotein inhibitors, inhibitors of NOS dephosphorylation, or by scavenging NO with hemoglobin or by increasing SOD activity to thereby reduce peroxynitrite anion formation [110]. Based on these studies, it was hypothesized that an increase in intracellular calcium by ischemia-induced NMDA receptor overactivation increases NO. NO also reportedly inhibits glutamate uptake and mediates the sustained opening of NMDA receptor ion channel [74, 111].

NO and Cerebral Ischemia

It is believed that constitutive NOS activity increases during ischemia due to a rise in intracellular Ca^{2+}. Constitutive NOS is activated by intracellular calcium concentrations slightly above the resting level and is maximally stimulated at 0.5 μM, suggesting that it is fully active during focal ischemia in which much higher levels are attained in neurons (10–100 μM) [29, 112]. This hypothesis is supported by demonstration of a striking increase in cortical NO levels from approximately 10 nM to 2.2μM within 3–24 min after middle cerebral artery (MCA) occlusion using a porphyrinic microsensor [113]. Brain nitrite (stable NO metabolite) and cGMP (a product of NO action) levels also rise within the first half hour of ischemia. These increases are effectively blocked by prior *L*-NA administration, indicating an enhanced NOS activity [114]. Electron paramagnetic resonance studies coupled with administering an in vivo spin-trap also demonstrate an increased NO level during ischemia [115]. A contribution of iNOS to the observed enhancement in NOS activity is unlikely since these effects were detected in the immediate period following MCA occlusion before induction of iNOS.

Up-regulation of nNOS and its mRNA also reportedly occurs, reaching a maximum in 4 h and continuing up to 7 days after permanent MCA occlusion [116]. However, available evidence suggests that constitutive NOS activity decreases shortly after its activation at the onset of ischemia [114]. A conformational change of the enzyme is likely because the decreased NOS activity was detected ex vivo where a controlled medium for pH, substrates and cofactors were optimally provided [114]. It should be noted that, with the available technology, the methods for detection of NO and NOS activity have limited spatial resolution. So, it is possible that NOS activity may differ between the core and penumbra. The penumbra, which has a residual oxygen supply, may be exposed to newly synthesized NO, especially during recurrent spreading depression waves [117]. However, even a short exposure to NO at the initial stage of ischemia may be sufficient to have a detrimental effect on neuronal survival by further deteriorating the already jeopardized cellular metabolism and/or damaging DNA. A similar argument has been raised for NMDA receptor-mediated neurotoxicity in ischemia because NMDA receptors are possibly inactivated after an initial overactivation during cerebral ischemia [118].

Neurons, perivascular nerves and cerebrovascular endothelium may form NO during cerebral ischemia. A late but sustained increase in NO levels may also occur due to expression of inducible NOS within microglia and invading inflammatory cells 24–72 h after the induction of ischemia [119, 120]. During the immediate period following ischemia, increased NO production in vascular endothelium or perivascular nerves may improve blood flow and be neuroprotective. Indeed, infusion of *L*-arginine, which dilates pial vessels via an NO-dependent mechanism and increases rCBF in normal as well as in ischemic brain, reduces infarct size [80, 81, 121] and leads to electrocorticogram recovery if blood flow enhancement exceeds the functional flow threshold of approximately 30% of pre-ischemic flow [122]. *L*-Arginine's effect on both blood flow and tissue protection is attenuated in parallel with a decrease in tissue NO production and NOS activity after ischemia [113, 114]. The NO-binding protein, guanylate cyclase, appears more robust and resistant to the effects of ischemia than NOS. Hence, intracarotid administration of NO donors leads to blood flow increases within the ischemic tissue for at least 1 h after arterial occlusion and a decrease in infarct size in models of focal ischemia [123]. In addition to its blood flow-enhancing effect, endothelial NO production may also improve microcirculation by reducing platelet aggregation and leukocyte adhesion [124–126].

Increases as well as reductions have been reported in the extent of tissue injury after *L*-NAME or *L*-NA administration in models of ischemia with MCA occlusion [for review, see 17]. On the basis of results showing that the NO precursor *L*-arginine decreases ischemic injury by enhancing blood flow in the peri-infarct area via NO-mediated mechanisms [80, 81, 121, 122], we postulated that nonselective inhibition of NO synthesis within vessels or platelets may obscure neuroprotective effects of NOS inhibition in nuerons during focal cerebral ischemia. In fact recent studies using selective nNOS inhibitors, 7-nitroindazole [59] or ARL-17477 [127] have reported neuroprotection. Using mutant mice that do not express the gene for the neuronal or endothelial isoforms of NOS, we have recently documented the detrimental role of neuro-

Table 1. Nitro-*L*-arginine's effect on infarct size 24 h after permanent MCA occlusion in the wild type (SV-129) and mutant mouse lacking expression of neuronal or endothelial isoforms of NOS

	Wild type	Mutants	
		nNOS (–)	eNOS (–)
Vehicle	large	small	very large
After *L*-NA	no change	large*	large*

*p<0.05 as compared to vehicle.

nal NO and the protective effect of endothelial NO on the development of cerebral infarction [18, 19] (table 1).

Brain NOS activity of nNOS knockouts was significantly reduced to less than 5% of the normal [128]. In line with this, low basal levels of cGMP and NO were found in mutant brains and no enhancement in cGMP and NO levels were observed during ischemia contrary to the robust increase in the wild type [18, 129]. The failure of neuronal NO production was associated with an increased resistance of mice to cerebral ischemia. The nNOS knockouts developed infarcts 38% smaller than the wild-type mice when subjected to 24-hour permanent MCA occlusion [18]. A decreased infarct size was also observed in mutants 3–4 days after permanent MCA occlusion. Neurological deficits were also less in nNOS knockout mice. Since reductions in regional cerebral blood within homologous ischemic regions after MCA occlusion were similar in both groups, the observed group differences were attributed to the consequence of neuronal NOS deletion but not due to hemodynamic factors. Administering nitro-*L*-arginine eliminated the resistance of nNOS knockouts to focal ischemic injury, presumably by eNOS inhibition, and its negative consequences on cerebral blood flow, leukocyte, and platelet function. eNOS appeared normally expressed in the endothelium of nNOS knockouts as detected both by immunohistochemistry and by a vasodilation response of pial arterioles to superfused acetylcholine at least equivalent to wild type [85, 86].

These data from mutant mice clearly demonstrate that lack of neuronal NOS gene expression is associated with reduced ischemic damage after MCA occlusion. Loss of perivascular nNOS activity could affect stroke hemodynamics unfavorably, however, it must have been compensated for by NO generated in endothelium and other mediators. In fact, nNOS knockout mice retain a normal cerebral vasodilatory response to hypercapnia and increased metabolism [85, 86]. The neuroprotective action obtained after deletion of neuronal NOS has also been demonstrated in mice subjected to 3 h of ischemia and 24 h of reperfusion. nNOS knockouts had a 69% smaller infarct size than wild-type mice [130]. Similar protection was measured after global ischemia [131]. In the latter study, fewer dead hippocampal neurons were counted 3 days after transient global ischemia induced by occluding both common carotid arteries plus basilar artery for 5 or 10 min. Not only were more hippocampal cells viable, but overall morbidity, weight loss, and neurological outcome was better in the mutant strain. NO has also been proposed as a neuroprotective agent when the redox state of the tissue favors the formation of NO^+, which inhibits NMDA receptor activity [52], or if NO scavenges superoxide and acts as an antioxidant [109]. However, these data from the nNOS knockouts also suggest that the cytotoxic effects of NO during focal ischemia exceed the proposed cytoprotective effects [52].

In line with the evidence from nNOS mutants, larger infarcts developed in eNOS knockout mice after 24-hour permanent MCA occlusion [19]. Deletion of eNOS rendered these mutants hypertensive, however, hypertension did not account for the increased susceptibility to ischemia because the infarct size did not decrease when hypertension was treated by hydralazine. Contrary to spontaneously hypertensive rats, no hypertensive changes were noted in the vessel wall or heart of these animals on preliminary histopathological analyses. However, possibly due to a reduced capacity of the cerebral arteries to adapt to hemodynamic changes (e.g., dilate), eNOS mutants developed more pronounced rCBF reductions in corresponding brain regions after MCA occlusion and exhibited proportionally lower rCBFs at reduced perfusion pressures during controlled hemorrhagic hypotension [19]. These unfavorable alterations in blood flow regulation in eNOS knockouts plus a likely enhancement in platelet and neutrophil adhesion may explain their sensitivity to ischemia. Unlike the nNOS mutant, *L*-NA administration decreased infarct size in the eNOS knockout mouse, presumably due to inhibition of the nNOS isoform and hence neuronal NO production that was shown to have detrimental consequences on ischemic neuronal death (table 1).

In conclusion, data from the mutant mice indicate that NO possesses a dual role in focal cerebral ischemia. Neuronal NO overproduction may be neurotoxic whereas endothelial NO may protect brain tissue by improving rCBF and other hemodynamic factors. These findings emphasize the need to develop selective inhibitors of the neuronal isoform to protect brain from injury.

Acknowledgments

Some of the studies described herein were supported by NIH grant NS10828, the MGH Interdepartmental Stroke Program Project, NS 26361, and an unrestricted research award in neuroscience from Bristol-Myers Squibb.

References

1 Marletta MA, Yoon PS, Ivengar R, Leaf CD, Whisnok JS: Macrophage oxidation of *L*-arginine to nitrite and nitrate: Nitric oxide is an intermediate. Biochemistry 1988;27:8706–8711.
2 Hibbs JB Jr, Taintor RR, Vavrin Z, Rachlin EM: Nitric oxide: A cytotoxic activated macrophage effector molecule. Biochem Biophys Res Commun 1988;157:87–94.
3 Palmer RMJ, Ferrige AG, Moncada S: Nitric oxide release accounts for the biological activity of endothelium-derived relaxing factor. Nature 1987;327:524–526.
4 Ignarro LJ, Buga GM, Wood KS, Byrns RE, Chaudhuri G: Endothelium-derived relaxing factor produced and released from artery and vein is nitric oxide. Proc Natl Acad Sci USA 1987;84: 9265–9269.
5 Moncada S, Higgs A: The *L*-arginine-nitric oxide pathway. N Engl J Med 1993;329:2002–2012.
6 Moncada S, Palmer RMJ, Higgs EA: Nitric oxide: Physiology, pathophysiology and pharmacology. Pharmacol Rev 1991;43:109–142.
7 Garthwaite J, Charles SL, Chess-Williams R: Endothelium-dependent relaxing factor release on activation of NMDA receptors suggests role for intercellular messenger in the brain. Nature 1988; 336:385–388.
8 Dawson TM, Snyder SH: Gases as biological messengers: Nitric oxide and carbon monoxide in the brain. J Neurosci 1994;14:5147–5159.
9 Knowles RG, Moncada S: Nitric oxide as a signal in blood vessels. Trends Biochem Sci 1992;17: 399–402.
10 Dawson TM, Dawson VL, Snyder SH: A novel neuronal messenger in brain: The free radical, nitric oxide. Ann Neurol 1992;32:297–311.
11 Gross SS, Wolin MS: Nitric oxide: Pathophysiological mechanisms. Annu Rev Physiol 1995;57: 737–769.
12 Marletta MA: Nitric oxide: Biosynthesis and biological significance. Trends Biochem Sci 1991;14: 488–492.
13 Bö L, Dawson TM, Wesselingh S, Mörk S, Choi S, Kong AP, Hanley D, Trapp BD: Induction of NOS in demyelinating regions of MS brain. Ann Neurol 1994;36:778–786.
14 Dawson VL, Dawson TM, Bartley DA, Uhl GR, Snyder SH: Mechanisms of nitric oxide mediated neurotoxicity in primary brain cultures. J Neurosci 1993;13:2651–2661.
15 Dawson VL, Dawson TM, London ED, Bredt DS, Snyder SH: Nitric oxide mediate glutamate neurotoxicity in primary cortical culture. Proc Natl Acad Sci USA 1991;88:6368–6371.
16 Dawson TM, Dawson VL: Nitric oxide: Actions and pathological roles. Neuroscientist 1995;1:7–18.
17 Dalkara T, Moskowitz MA: Complex role of nitric oxide in cerebral ischemia. Brain pathol 1994; 4:49–57.
18 Huang Z, Huang PL, Panahian N, Dalkara T, Fishman MC, Moskowitz MA: Effects of cerebral ischemia in mice deficient in neuronal nitric oxide synthase. Science 1994;265:1883–1885.
19 Huang Z, Huang PL, J Ma, Meng W, Ayata C, Fishman MC, Moskowitz MA: Enlarged infarcts in endothelial nitric oxide synthase knockout mice are attenuated by nitro-*L*-arginine. J Cereb Blood Flow Metab 1996;16:981–987.
20 Griffith OW, Stuehr DJ: Nitric oxide synthases: Properties and catalytic mechanism. Annu Rev Physiol 1995;57:707–736.
21 Bredt DS, Snyder SH: Isolation of nitric oxide synthase, a calmodulin-requiring enzyme. Proc Natl Acad Sci USA 1990;87:682–685.

22 Hevel JM, White KA, Marletta MA: Purification of the inducible murine macrophage nitric oxide synthase: Identification as a flavoprotein. J Biol Chem 1991;266:22789–22791.
23 Pollock JS, Forstermann U, Mitchell JA, Warner TD, Schmidt HHHW, Nakane M, Murad F: Purification and characterization of particulate endothelium-derived relaxing factor synthase from cultured and native bovine aortic endothelial cells. Proc Natl Acad Sci USA 1991;88:10480–10484.
24 Geller DA, Lowenstein CJ, Shapiro RA, Nussler AK, DiSilvio M, Wang SC, Nakayama DK, Simmons RL, Snyder SH, Billar TR: Molecular cloning and expression of inducible nitric oxide synthase from human hepatocytes. Proc Natl Acad Sci USA 1993;90:3491–3493.
25 Charles IG, Palmer MJ, Hickery MS, Bayliss MT, Chubb AP, Hall VS, Moss DW, Moncada S: Cloning, characterization and expression of a cDNA encoding an inducible nitric oxide synthase from the human chondrocyte. Proc Natl Acad Sci USA 1993;90:11419–11423.
26 Bredt DS, Hwang PM, Glatt CE, Lowenstein C, Reed RR, Snyder SH: Cloned and expressed nitric oxide synthase structurally resembles P-450 reductase. Nature 1991;351:714–718.
27 Bredt DS, Glatt EC, Hwang PM, Fotuhi M, Dawson TM, Snyder SH: Nitric oxide synthase protein mRNA discretely localized in neuronal populations of the mammalian CNS together with NADPH diaphorase. Neuron 1991;7:615–624.
28 Dinerman JL, Dawson TM, Schell MJ, Snowman A, Snyder SH: Endothelial nitric oxide synthase localized to hippocampal pyramidal cells: Implications for synaptic plasticity. Proc Natl Acad Sci USA 1994;91:4214–4218.
29 Knowles RG, Palacios M, Palmer RMJ, Moncada S: Formation of nitric oxide from *L*-arginine in the central nervous system: A transduction mechanism for stimulation of the soluble guanylate cyclase. Proc Natl Acad Sci USA 1989;86:5159–5162.
30 Cho HJ, Xie QW, Calaycay J, Mumford RA, Swiderek KM, Lee TD, Nathan C: Calmodulin as a tightly bound subunit of calcium-calmodulin independent nitric oxide synthase. J Exp Med 1992; 176:599–604.
31 Bredt DS, Hwang PM, Snyder SH: Localization of nitric oxide synthase indicating a neural role for nitric oxide. Nature 1990;347:768–770.
32 Nozaki K, Moskowitz MA, Maynard KI, Koketsu N, Dawson TM, Bredt DS, Snyder SH: Possible origin and distribution of immunoreactive nitric oxide synthase-containing nerve fibers in cerebral arteries. J Cereb Blood Flow Metab 1993;13:70–79.
33 Murphy S, Simmons ML, Agullo L, Garcia A, Feinstein DL, Galea E, Reis DJ, Minc-Golomb D, Schwartz JP: Synthesis of nitric oxide in CNS glial cells. Trends Neurosci 1993;16:323–328.
34 Burnett AL, Lowenstein CJ, Bredt DS, Cheng TSK, Snyder SH: Nitric oxide: A physiological mediator of penile erection. Science 1992;257:401–403.
35 Knowles RG, Salter M, Brooks SL, Moncada S: Anti-inflammatory glucocorticoids inhibit the induction by endotoxin of nitric oxide synthase in the lung, liver and aorta of the rat. Biochem Biophys Res Commun 1990;172:1042–1048.
36 Gross SS, Jaffe EA, Levi R, Kilbourn RG: Cytokine-activated endothelial cells express an isotype of nitric oxide synthase which is tetrahydrobiopterin-dependent, calmodulin-independent and inhibited by arginine analogs with a rank-order potency characteristic of activated macrophages. Biochem Biophys Res Commun 1991;178:823–829.
37 Chao CC, Hu S, Molitor TW, Shaskan EG, Peterson PK: Activated microglia mediate neuronal cell injury via a nitric oxide mechanism. J Immunol 1992;149:2736–2741.
38 Nakane M, Schmidt HHHW, Pollock JS, Forstermann U, Murad F: Cloned human brain nitric oxide synthase is highly expressed in skeletal muscle. FEBS Lett 1993;316:175–180.
39 Marsden PA, Heng HHQ, Scherer SW, Stewart RJ, Hall AV, Shi XM, Tsui LC, Schappert KT: Structural and chromosomal localization of the human constitutive endothelial nitric oxide synthase gene. J Biol Chem 1993;268:17478–17488.
40 Xu W, Charles IG, Moncada S, Gorman P, Sheer D, Liu L, Emson P: Mapping of the genes encoding human inducible and endothelial NOS to the pericentric region of chromosome 17 and to chromosome 7, respectively. Genomics 1994;21:419–422.
41 Garthwaite J, Boulton CL: Nitric oxide signaling in the central nervous system. Annu Rev Physiol 1995;57:683–706.

42 Stamler JS, Simon DI, Osborne JA, Mullins ME, Jaraki O, Michel T, Singel DJ, Loscalzo J: S-nitrosylation of proteins by nitric oxide: Synthesis and characterization of novel biologically active compounds. Proc Natl Acad Sci USA 1992;89:444–448.

43 Marletta MA: Mammalian synthesis of nitrite, nitrate, nitric oxide and N-nitrosating agents. Chem Res Toxicol 1988;1:249–257.

44 Beckman JS, Chen J, Conger K: The importance of superoxide in nitric oxide-dependent cerebral ischemic injury; in Moskowitz MA, Kaplan LR (eds): Cerebrovascular Diseases. Newton, Butterworth-Heinemann, 1995, pp 25–36.

45 Griscavage JM, Rogers NE, Sherman MP, Ignarro LJ: Inducible nitric oxide synthase from rat alveolar macrophage cell line is inhibited by nitric oxide. J Immunol 1993;151:6329–6337.

46 Olson DR, Kon C, Breckenridge BM: Calcium ion effects on guanylate cyclase of brain. Life Sci 1976;18:935–940.

47 Ignarro LJ, Kadowitz PJ: The pharmacological and physiological role of cyclic GMP in vascular smooth muscle relaxation. Annu Rev Pharmacol Toxicol 1985;25:171–191.

48 Ahlner J, Anderson RGG, Torfgard K, Axelson KL: Organic nitrate esters: Clinical use and mechanisms of actions. Pharmacol Rev 1991;43:351–423.

49 Salvemini D, Misko TP, Masferrer JL, Seibert K, Currie MG, Needleman P: Nitric oxide activates cyclooxygenase enzymes. Proc Natl Acad Sci USA 1993;90:7240–7244.

50 Brune B, Dimmeler S, Molina-y-Vedia L, Lapetina EG: Nitric oxide: A signal for ADP-ribosylation of proteins. Life Sci 1994;54:61–70.

51 Stamler JS, Singel DJ, Loscalzo J: Biochemistry of nitric oxide and its redox-activated forms. Science 1992;258:1898–1902.

52 Lipton SA, Choi Y, Pan Z, Lei SZ, Chen HV, Sucher NJ, Loscalzo J, Singel DJ, Stamler J: A redox-based mechanism for the neuroprotective and neurodestructive effects of nitric oxide and related nitroso-compounds. Nature 1993;364:626–632.

53 Moore PK, al-Swayeh OA, Chong NWS, Evans R, Mirzazadeh S, Gibson A: *L*-N^G-nitroarginine, a novel, *L*-arginine-reversible inhibitor of endothelium-dependent vasodilation in vivo. Br J Pharmacol 1990;99:408–412.

54 Rees DD, Palmer RMJ, Schulz R, Hodson F, Moncada S: Characterization of three inhibitors of endothelial nitric oxide synthase in vitro and in vivo. Br J Pharmacol 1990;101:746–752.

55 Dwyer MA, Bredt DS, Snyder SH: Nitric oxide synthase: Irreversible inhibition by *L*-N^G-nitroarginine in brain in vitro and in vivo. Biochem Biophys Res Commun 1991;176:1136–1141.

56 Ogden JE, Moore PK: Inhibition of nitric oxide synthase – potential for a novel class of therapeutic agent. Trend Biol Tech 1995;13:70–78.

57 Lambert LE, Whitten JP, Baron BM, Chang HC, Doherty NS, McDonald JH: Nitric oxide in the CNS, endothelium and macrophages differ in its sensitivity to inhibition by arginine analogs. Life Sci 1991;48:69–75.

58 Moore PK, Wallace P, Gaffen Z, Hart SL, Babbedge RC: Characterization of a novel nitric oxide synthase inhibitor 7-nitroindazole and related indazoles: Antinociceptive and cardiovascular effects. Br J Pharmacol 1993;110:219–224.

59 Yoshida T, Limmroth V, Irikura K, Moskowitz M: The NOS inhibitor 7-nitroindazole decreases focal infarct volume but not the response to topical acetylcholine in pial vessels. J Cereb Blood Flow Metab 1994;14:924–929.

60 Babbedge RC, Bland-Ward SL, Hart SL, Moore PK: Inhibition of rat cerebellar nitric oxide synthase by 7-nitroindazole and related substituted indazoles. Br J Pharmacol 1993;110:225–228.

61 Moore WM, Webber RK, Jerome GM, Tjoeng FS, Misko TP, Currie MG: 5-N6-(1-iminoethyl)lysine: A selective inhibitor of inducible nitric oxide synthase. J Med Chem 1994;37:3886–3888.

62 Furfins ES, Harmon MF, Paith JE, Knowles RG, Salter M, Kiff RJ, Duffy C, Hazelwood R, Oplinger JA, Garvey EP: Potent and selective inhibition of human nitric oxide synthases: Selective inhibition of neuronal nitric oxide synthase by S-methyl-*L*-thiocitrulline and S-ethyl-*L*-thiocitrulline. J Biol Chem 1994;269:26677–26683.

63 Misko TP, Moore WM, Kasten TP, Nickols GA, Corbet JA: Selective inhibition of inducible nitric oxide synthase by aminoguanidine. Eur J Pharmacol 1993;233:119–125.

64 Buxton IL, Cheek DJ, Eckman D, Westfall DP, Sanders KM, Keef KD: N^G-nitro-*L*-arginine methyl ester of arginine are muscarinic antagonists. Circ Res 1993;72:1374–1380.

65 Peterson DA, Peterson DC, Archer S, Weir EK: The non specificity of specific nitric oxide synthase inhibitors. Biochem Biophys Res Commun 1992;187:797–801.

66 Bogle RG, Moncada S, Pearson JD, Mann GE: Identification of inhibitors of nitric oxide synthase that do not interact with endothelial cell *L*-arginine transporter. Br J Pharmacol 1992;105:768–770.

67 Hecker DR: Pressure-induced myogenic activation of cat cerebral arteries is dependent on intact endothelium. Circ Res 1987;60:102–107.

68 Fukuto JM, Chaudhuri G: Inhibition of constitutive and inducible nitric oxide synthase: Potential selective inhibition. Annu Rev Pharmacol Toxicol 1995;35:165–194.

69 Gally JA, Montague PR, Reeke GN Jr, Edelman GM: The NO hypothesis: Possible effects of a short-lived rapidly diffusible signal in the development and function of the nervous system. Proc Natl Acad Sci USA 1990;87:3547–3551.

70 O'Dell TJ, Hawkins RD, Kandel E, Arancio O: Tests of the roles of two diffusible substances in long-term potentiation: Evidence for nitric oxide as a possible early retrograde messenger. Proc Natl Acad Sci USA 1991;88:11285–11289.

71 O'Dell TJ, Huang PL, Dawson TM, Dinerman JL, Snyder SH, Kandel ER, Fishman MC: Endothelial NOS and the blockade of LTP by NOS inhibitors in mice lacking neuronal NOS. Science 1994; 265:542–546.

72 Pape HC, Mager R: Nitric oxide controls oscillatory activity in thalamocortical neurons. Neuron 1992;9:441–448.

73 Desole MS, Kim WK, Rabin RA, Laychock SG: Nitric oxide reduces depolarization-induced calcium influx in PC12 cells by a cyclic GMP-mediated mechanism. Neuropharmacology 1994;33:193–198.

74 Pogun S, Dawson V, Kuhar MJ: Nitric oxide inhibits ^{3}H-glutamate transport in synaptosomes. Synapse 1994;18:21–26.

75 Rivier C, Shen GH: In the rat, endogenous nitric oxide modulates the response of the hypothalamic-pituitary-adrenal axis to interleukin-1β, vasopressin and oxytocin. J Neurosci 1994;14:1985–1993.

76 Faraci FM: Role of nitric oxide in regulation of basilar artery tone. Am J Physiol 1990;259: H1216–H1221.

77 Busija DW, Leffler CW, Wagerle LC: Mono-*L*-arginine-containing compounds dilate piglet arterioles via an endothelium-derived relaxing factor-like substance. Circ Res 1990;67:1374–1380.

78 Tanaka K, Gotoh F, Gomi S, Takashima S, Mihara B, Shirai T, Nogawa S, Nagata E: Inhibition of nitric oxide synthesis induces a significant reduction in local cerebral blood flow in the rat. Neurosci Lett 1991;127:129–132.

79 Faraci FM, Brian JE: Nitric oxide and the cerebral circulation. Stroke 1994;25:692–703.

80 Morikawa E, Rosenblatt S, Moskowitz MA: *L*-Arginine dilates rat pial arterioles by nitric oxide-dependent mechanisms and increases blood flow during focal cerebral ischemia. Br J Pharmacol 1992;107:905–907.

81 Morikawa E, Moskowitz MA, Huang Z, Yoshida T, Irikura K, Dalkara T: *L*-Arginine infusion promotes nitric oxide-dependent vasodilation, increases regional cerebral blood flow, and reduces infarction volume in the rat. Stroke 1994;25:429–435.

82 Iadecola C, Pelligrino DA, Moskowitz MA, Lassen NA: Nitric oxide synthase inhibition and cerebrovascular regulation. J Cereb Blood Flow Metab 1994;14:175–192.

83 Pelligrino DA, Koenig HM, Albrecht RF: Nitric oxide synthesis and regional cerebral blood flow responses to hypercapnia and hypoxia in the rat. J Cereb Blood Flow Metab 1993;13:80–87.

84 Irikura K, Maynard KI, Lee WS, Moskowitz MA: *L*-Nitroarginine decreases cortical hyperemia and brain cGMP levels following CO_2 inhalation in Sprague-Dawley rats. Am J Physiol 1994;267: H837–H843.

85 Irikura K, Huang PL, Ma J, Lee WS, Dalkara T, Fishman MC, Dawson TM, Snyder SH, Moskowitz MA: Cerebrovascular alterations in mice lacking neuronal nitric oxide synthase gene expression. Proc Natl Acad Sci USA 1995;92:6823–6827.

86 Ma J, Ayata C, Huang P, Fishman MC, Moskowitz MA: Regional cerebral blood flow response to vibrissal stimulation in mice lacking type I NOS gene expression. Am J Physiol 1996;270: H1085–H1090.

87 Ayata C, Ma J, Meng W, Huang P, Moskowitz MA: *L*-NA-sensitive rCBF augmentation during vibrissal stimulation in type III nitric oxide synthase mutant mice. J Cereb Blood Flow Metab 1996; 16:539–541.
88 Faraci FM, Breese RR: Nitric oxide mediates vasodilation in response to activation of N-methyl-*D*-aspartate receptors in brain. Circ Res 1993;72:476–480.
89 Colona DM, Meng W, Deal DD, Busija DW: Nitric oxide promotes arteriolar dilation during cortical spreading depression in rabbits. Stroke 1994;25:2463-2470.
90 Koh J, Choi DW: Vulnerability of cultured cortical neurons to damage by excitotoxins: Differential susceptibility of neurons containing NADPH-diaphorase. J Neurosci 1988;8:2153–2163.
91 Uemura Y, Kowall NW, Beal MF: Selective sparing of NADPH-diaphorase-somatostatin-neuropeptide Y neurons in ischemic gerbil striatum. Ann Neurol 1990;27:620–625.
92 Fischer HC, Kuljis RO: Multiple types of nitrogen monoxide synthase-/NADPH-diaphorase containing neurons in the human cerebral neocortex. Brain Res 1994;654:105–117.
93 Kwon NS, Stuehr DJ, Nathan CF: Inhibition of tumor cell ribonucleotide reductase by macrophage-derived nitric oxide. J Exp Med 1991;174:761–767.
94 Liu RH, Hotchkiss JH: Potential genotoxicity of chronically elevated nitric oxide: A review. Mutat Res 1995;339:73–89.
95 Zhang J, Dawson VL, Dawson TM, Snyder SH: Nitric oxide activation of poly(ADP-ribose) synthase in neurotoxicity. Science 1994;263:686–689.
96 Blanco FJ, Ochs RL, Schwarz H, Lotz M: Chondrocyte apoptosis induced by nitric oxide. Am J Pathol 1995;146:75–85.
97 Kitajima I, Kawahara K, Nakajima T, Soejima Y, Matsuyama T, Maruyama I: Nitric oxide-mediated apoptosis in murine mastocytoma. Biochem Biophys Res Commun 1994;204:244–251.
98 Messmer UK, Lapetina EG, Brune B: Nitric oxide-induced apoptosis in RAW 264.7 macrophages is antagonized by protein kinase C- and protein kinase A-activating compounds. Mol Pharmacol 1995;47:757–765.
99 Heron A, Pollard H, Dessi F, Moreau J, Lasbennes F, Ben-Ari Y, Charriaut-Marlangue C: Regional variability in DNA fragmentation after global ischemia evidenced by combined histological and gel electrophoresis observations in the rat brain. J Neurochem 1993;61:1973–1976.
100 MacManus J, Hill I, Huang Z, Rasquinha I, Xue D, Buchan A: DNA damage consistent with apoptosis in transient focal ischemic neocortex. Neuroreport 1994;5:493–496.
101 Tominiga T, Kure S, Narisawa K, Yoshimoto T: Endonuclease activation following focal ischemic injury in the rat brain. Brain Res 1993;608:21–26.
102 Charriaut-Marlangue C, Margaill I, Plotkine M, Ben-Ari Y: Early endonuclease activation following reversible focal ischemia in the rat brain. J Cereb Blood Flow Metab 1995;15:385–388.
103 Li Y, Chopp M, Jiang N, Yao F, Zaloga C: Temporal profile of in situ DNA fragmentation after middle cerebral artery occlusion in the rat. J Cereb Blood Flow Metab 1995;15:389–397.
104 Beckman JS: The double-edged role of nitric oxide in the brain function and superoxide-mediated injury. J Dev Physiol 1991;15:53–59.
105 Koppenol WH, Moreno JJ, Pryor WA, Ischiropoulos H, Beckman JS: Peroxynitrite, a cloaked oxidant formed by nitric oxide and superoxide. Chem Res Toxicol 1992;5:834–842.
106 Beckman JS: Peroxynitrite versus hydroxyl radical: The role of nitric oxide in superoxide-dependent cerebral injury. Ann NY Acad Sci 1994;738:69–75.
107 Pou S, Pou WS, Bredt DS, Snyder SH, Rosen GM: Generation of superoxide by brain nitric oxide synthase. J Biol Chem 1992;267:24137–24141.
108 Kanner J, Harel S, Granit R: Nitric oxide as an antioxidant. Arch Biochem Biophys 1991;289: 130–136.
109 Niu XF, Smith CW, Kubes P: Intracellular oxidative stress induced by nitric oxide synthesis inhibition increases endothelial cell adhesion to neutrophils. Circ Res 1994;74:1133–1140.
110 Dawson VL, Dawson TM, Bartley DA, Uhl GR, Snyder SH: Mechanisms of nitric oxide mediated neurotoxicity in primary brain cultures. J Neurosci 1993;13:2651–2661.
111 Akira T, Henry B, Wasterlain CG: Nitric oxide mediates the sustained opening of NMDA receptor-gated ionic channels which follows transient excitotoxic exposure in hippocampal slices. Brain Res 1994;652:190–194.

112 Silver IA, Erecinska M: Intracellular and extracellular (Ca^{2+}) in hypoxia and ischemia in rat brain in vivo. J Gen Physiol 1990;95:837–866.
113 Malinski T, Bailey F, Zhang ZG, Chopp M: Nitric oxide measured by a porphyrinic microsensor in rat brain after transient middle cerebral artery occlusion. J Cereb Blood Flow Metab 1993;13:355–358.
114 Kader A, Frazzini VI, Solomon RA, Trifiletti RR: Nitric oxide production during focal cerebral ischemia. Stroke 1993;24:1709–1716.
115 Sato S, Tominaga T, Ohnishi T, Ohnishi ST: EPR spin-trapping study of nitric oxide formation during bilateral carotid occlusion in the rat. Biochim Biophys Acta 1993;1181:195–197.
116 Zhang ZG, Chopp M, Gautam S, Zaloga C, Chang RL, Schmidt HHHW, Pollock JS, Förstermann U: Upregulation of neuronal nitric oxide synthase and mRNA, and selective sparing of nitric oxide synthase-containing neurons after focal cerebral ischemia in rat. Brain Res 1994;654:85–95.
117 Gill R, Andine P, Hillered L, Persson L, Hagberg H: The effect of MK-801 on cortical spreading depression in the penumbral zone following focal ischemia in the rat. J Cereb Blood Flow Metab 1992;12:371–379.
118 Dalkara T, Ayata C, Demirci M, Erdemli G, Onur R: Effects of cerebral ischemia on NMDA and dihydropyridine-sensitive calcium currents. Stroke 1996;27:127–133.
119 Iadecola C, Xu X, Zhang F, el-Fakahany EE, Ross ME: Marked induction of calcium-independent nitric oxide synthase activity after focal cerebral ischemia. J Cereb Blood Flow Metab 1995;15:52–59.
120 Iadecola C, Zhang F, Xu S, Casey R, Ross ME: Inducible nitric oxide synthase gene expression in brain following cerebral ischemia. J Cereb Blood Flow Metab 1995;15:378–384.
121 Morikawa E, Huang Z, Moskowitz MA: *L*-Arginine decreases infarct size caused by middle cerebral arterial occlusion in SHR. Am J Physiol 1992;263:H1632–H1635.
122 Dalkara T, Morikawa H, Moskowitz MA, Panahian N: Blood flow-dependent functional recovery in a rat model of cerebral ischemia. Am J Physiol 1994;267:H837–H838.
123 Zhang F, White JG, Iadecola C: Nitric oxide donors increase blood flow and reduce brain damage in focal cerebral ischemia: Evidence that nitric oxide is beneficial in the early stages of cerebral ischemia. J Cereb Blood Flow Metab 1994;14:217–226.
124 Rosenblum WI, Nishimura H, Ellis EF, Nelson GH: The endothelium-dependent effects of thimerosal on mouse pial arterioles in vivo: Evidence for control of microvascular events by EDRF as well as prostaglandins. J Cereb Blood Flow Metab 1992;12:703–706.
125 Garcia JH, Yoshida Y, Chen H, Li Y, Zhang ZG, Lian J, Chen S, Chopp M: Progression from ischemic injury to infarct following middle cerebral artery occlusion in the rat. Am J Pathol 1993; 142:623–635.
126 Kurose I, Wolf R, Grisham MB, Granger DN: Modulation of ischemia/reperfusion-induced microvascular dysfunction by nitric oxide. Circ Res 1994;74:376–382.
127 Zhang ZG, Reif D, Macdonald J, Tang WX, Kamp DK, Gentile RJ, Shakespeare WC, Murray RJ, Chopp M: ARL 17477, a potent and selective neuronal NOS inhibitor decreases infarct volume after transient middle cerebral artery occlusion in rats. J Cereb Blood Flow Metab 1996;16:599–604.
128 Huang PL, Dawson TM, Bredt DS, Snyder SH, Fishman MC: Targeted disruption of neuronal nitric oxide synthase gene. Cell 1993;75:1773–1786.
129 Mullins ME, Sondheimer NJ, Huang Z, Singel DJ, Stamler J, Huang PL, Fishman MC, Moskowitz MA: nNOS-deficient mice are able to produce nitric oxide activity in cortical tissue as measured by ESR NO˙ quantification. In preparation.
130 Hara H, Huang PL, Panahian N, Fishman MC, Moskowitz MA: Reduced brain edema and infarction volume in mice lacking the neuronal isoform of nitric oxide synthase after transient MCA occlusion. J Cereb Blood Flow Metab 1996;16:605–611.
131 Panahian N, Yoshida T, Huang PL, Hedley-Whyte ET, Dalkara T, Fishman MC, Moskowitz MA: Attenuated hippocampal damage after global cerebral ischemia in mice mutant in neuronal nitric oxide synthase. Neuroscience 1996;72:343–354.

Michael A. Moskowitz, MD, Stroke and Neurovascular Regulation Laboratory,
Department of Neurology and Neurosurgical Service, Massachusetts General Hospital,
Harvard Medical School, 149 13th Street, Room 6403, Charlestown, MA 02129 (USA)

Hsu CY (ed): Ischemic Stroke: From Basic Mechanisms to New Drug Development.
Monogr Clin Neurosci. Basel, Karger, 1998, vol 16, pp 46–64

Inflammatory Response and Adhesion Molecules in Focal Cerebral Ischemia

Zheng Gang Zhang[a], *Michael Chopp*[b]

[a] Henry Ford Health Science Center, Neurology Department, Detroit, Mich., and
[b] Oakland University, Physics Department, Rochester, Mich., USA

Documentation of inflammatory cell response to injury in the central nervous system (CNS) has a long history [1–3]. However, only in the last decade, with identification of specific cell adhesion and chemoattractant molecules, have the molecular mechanisms underlying leukocyte endothelial cell adhesion been uncovered. Recruitment of blood leukocytes into ischemic tissue involves a well-coordinated and dynamic sequence of events in which at least three families of cell adhesion molecules and chemoattractant molecules play a central role in leukocyte-endothelial interactions: the selectins, the integrins, the immunoglobulin superfamily and chemoattractants [4–7]. These molecules act in an orchestrated sequence to facilitate the leukocyte-endothelial cell adhesion cascade. The initial event in this cascade is that of selectin-mediated leukocyte rolling. Subsequently, chemoattractant molecules, such as interleukin-8 (IL-8) and monocyte chemoattractant protein-1 (MCP-1) activate integrin adhesiveness. Integrin, such as macrophage antigen-1 (Mac-1), expression on the surface of neutrophils can be dramatically up-regulated by chemoattractant stimulated fusion of secretory granules with the cytoplasmic membrane. An immunoglobulin superfamily member, such as intercellular adhesion molecule-1 (ICAM-1), then binds the integrin and causes leukocytes to firmly adhere to the endothelium. As a consequence of the progress made in understanding the molecular mediators of leukocyte-endothelial cell interaction and the identification of families of adhesion molecules, new therapeutic interventions directed towards the blocking of one or more of the steps in the leukocyte-endothelial adhesion cascade have been successfully employed to reduce inflammatory cell-mediated damage in experimental ischemia/reperfusion injury in heart [8], liver [9], kidney [10], lung [11], spinal cord [12] and brain [13].

This chapter begins with a brief review of the temporal profile of both exogenous (leukocytes) and endogenous (microglia) inflammatory response after focal cerebral ischemia. This is followed by a description of recent studies concerning the expression of adhesion and chemoattractant molecules in focal cerebral ischemia and associated therapeutic approaches to block leukocyte, particularly neutrophil, endothelial adhesion and thereby to reduce ischemic cell damage. Experimental data implicating factors that may mediate expression of adhesion molecules after focal cerebral ischemia are also provided.

Temporal Profile of Inflammatory Response

Accumulation of polymorphonuclear leukocytes (PMNL) and monocytes has been demonstrated after clinical and experimental stroke since the 1970s. Sörnās et al. [2] were among the first investigators to provide evidence of the participation of leukocytes in human stroke. Cytological examination of cerebrospinal fluid samples obtained from patients after stroke revealed that accumulation of PMNL in cerebrospinal fluid was maximal 48–72 h after the onset of stroke. Using static brain scintigraphy and indium-111-labeled leukocytes, Pozzilli et al. [14] demonstrated leukocyte accumulation in human cerebral infarcts 2–14 days after the onset of stroke symptoms. Delayed and long-lasting leukocyte accumulation in human stroke is further supported by a recent study using technetium-99m hexamethylpropyleneamine oxine-labeled leukocyte brain single-photon emission computed tomography [15]. Leukocyte accumulation in areas of perfusion defect persisted 1–5 weeks after acute hemispheric ischemic stroke.

An early study in a primate model of permanent middle cerebral artery (MCA) occlusion revealed that PMNL accumulation was maximal at 48–72 h after onset of ischemia [3]. However, the first evidence of early accumulation of PMNL in cerebral ischemia resulted from the work of Hallenbeck et al. [16]. PMNL were shown to progressively accumulate in areas of low cerebral blood flow (CBF) during the first 4 h of reperfusion in a dog model of cerebral air embolism. The early presence of PMNL in focal cerebral ischemia has been subsequently confirmed in a series of experiments of MCA occlusion by histopathology and myeloperoxidase (MPO) activity assay. del Zoppo et al. [17] demonstrated that PMNL blocked approximately 8% of brain microvessels in the hypoperfused region of the MCA territory in a primate model of 3 h of MCA occlusion and 1 h of reperfusion. These studies suggest that PMNL contribute to perfusion deficits after transient focal cerebral ischemia.

Using a modified MPO activity assay, Barone et al. [18] first quantitated PMNL accumulation in the ischemic brain after permanent MCA occlusion

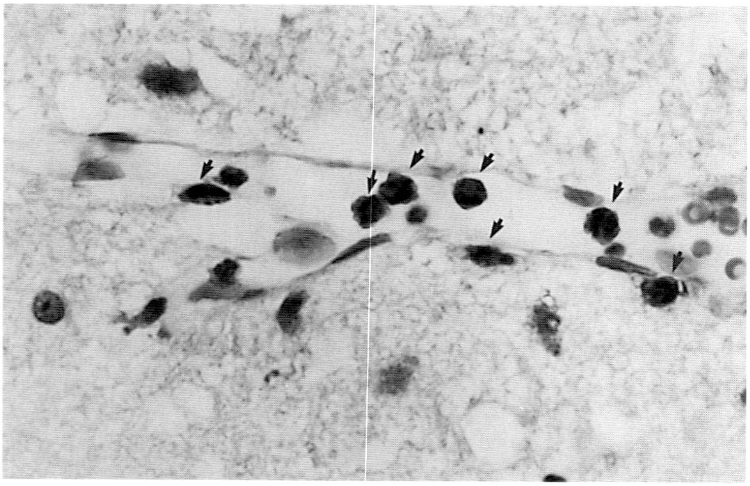

Fig. 1. Photomicrograph of MPO-immunoreactive neutrophils in a cerebral vessel and in the parenchyma obtained from a rat subjected to 2 h of MCA occlusion and 10 h of reperfusion.

in spontaneous hypertensive rats (SHR). A significant increase in MPO activity was found in the ischemic cortex 24 h after MCA occlusion. The same group also recently showed that transient (160 min) MCA occlusion resulted in a significant increase in MPO activity in ischemic tissue as early as 6 h after reperfusion, while a significant increase of MPO activity in the ischemic cortex was observed 12 h after permanent MCA occlusion in SHR [19]. The time course of postischemic PMNL and monocyte accumulation has been documented in Wistar rats after focal cerebral ischemia produced by occlusion of MCA with a nylon monofilament. Histopathology (light and electron microscopy), and MPO immunohistochemistry revealed early PMNL accumulation in the cerebral microvessels at 1 h of MCA occlusion and in the parenchyma at 1 h of reperfusion after 2 h of MCA occlusion [20, 21]. Figure 1 shows MPO immunoreactive neutrophils in a cerebral vessel and in the parenchyma obtained from a rat subjected to 2 h of MCA occlusion and 10 h of reperfusion. The number of PMNL maximized at 48 h and 72 h after transient (2 h) and permanent MCA occlusion [22], respectively. These data suggest that reperfusion promotes earlier PMNL migration into the parenchyma than does permanent MCA occlusion.

In addition to the accumulation of PMNL, monocytes and macrophages are present in brain after focal cerebral ischemia. Monocytes were observed at 12 h after permanent MCA occlusion in rats [20]. A large number of monocytes and macrophages accumulate in the ischemic brain 24 h and persist to 168 h after MCA occlusion [20, 22]. Monocytes and macrophages persist up to 60 days in photochemically induced ischemia of the rat cortex [23].

Microglial response is robust after global and focal cerebral ischemia in the rat [24–27]. The morphology of microglia changes from ramified to ameboid when they are stimulated [28]. Ameboid microglia produce interleukin-1β (IL-1β) as well as other cytokines [29, 30]. Using lectin histochemistry with the B4-isolectin from *Griffonia simplicifolia*, we found that ameboid-like microglia were present in the ischemic lesion between 2 and 10 h of reperfusion in rats subjected to 2 h of MCA occlusion (fig. 2). Ameboid cells became predominant in the ischemic core of the lesion at 22 h of reperfusion [31]. Based on morphology alone, we cannot distinguish between ameboid-shaped microglia and infiltrating monocyte-derived macrophages. Lymphocytes are also present within the ischemic brain after MCA occlusion. A detailed temporal profile lymphocyte accumulation has recently been performed in photochemically induced focal cerebral lesion in the rat [23]. T lymphocyte (CD5+) accumulation was observed in the subpial and cortical vessels at 1 and 2 days, peaked at 3–7 days and persisted to 30 days after photothrombosis.

The above studies suggest that leukocytes are present in ischemic or injured cerebral tissue and may contribute to ischemic neuronal damage. Two proposed mechanisms of leukocyte contribution to pathogenesis after cerebral ischemia are: (1) reduction of CBF by direct microvascular occlusion after leukocytes adhere to endothelium [32]; and (2) exacerbation of microcirculation and neuronal injury via oxygen radical production, proteases, cytokines etc. released by leukocytes [1, 33]. Therefore, it is reasonable to attempt to reduce the accumulation of leukocytes within the ischemic area and consequently to reduce the ischemic cell damage. Depletion of PMNL, using mechlorethamine [34], antiserum [35, 36] or antibody [37] against neutrophils in animal models of cerebral ischemia and reperfusion, confirms the contribution of leukocytes to oxygen radical production, postischemic hypoperfusion, brain edema, and ischemic cell damage. However, the induction of neutropenia is not an optimal way to reduce postischemic inflammatory response because neutropenia causes a reduction of other inflammatory cells, and secondary pathophysiological events resulting from neutropenia may complicate and obscure the singular contribution of neutrophils or other inflammatory cells to the ongoing process of ischemic cell damage. New therapeutic approaches directed to block the molecules involved in promoting leukocyte-endothelial adhesion have been performed in experimental focal cerebral ischemia and will be described.

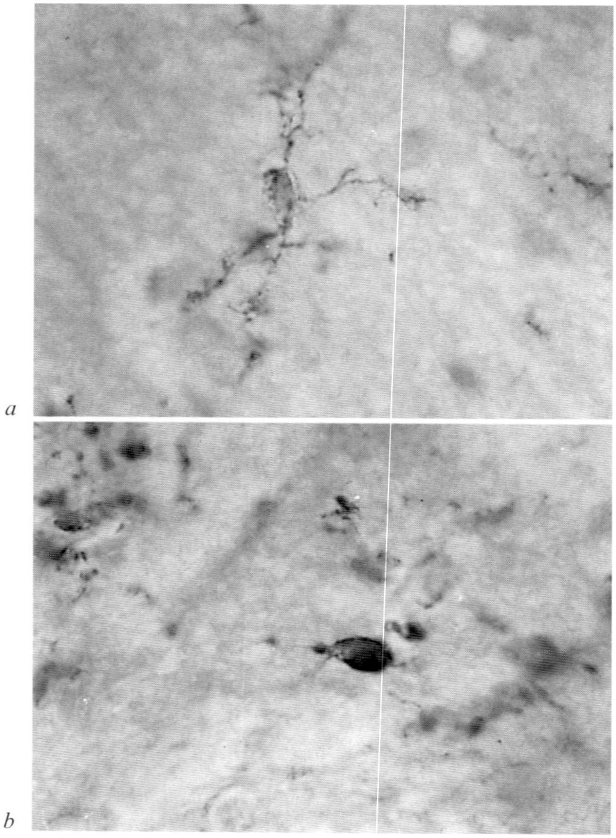

Fig. 2. Photomicrographs of B_4-isolectin-stained microglia: (*a*) a ramified microglial cell in the cortex obtained from a rat without ischemia and (*b*) an ameboid-like microglial cell in the ischemic cortex at 4 h of reperfusion after 2 h of MCA occlusion.

Selectins

At sites of tissue injury and inflammation the selectin family of adhesion molecules mediates the initial attachment of leukocytes to endothelial cells prior to their firm adhesion and subsequent diapedesis [38, 39]. The selectin family consists of three closely related cell surface molecules: L-selectin (CD62L), E-selectin (CD62E) and P-selectin (CD62P). L-selectin is expressed on all circulating leukocytes, except for a subpopulation of lymphocytes [40]. P-selectin is stored in the Weibel-Palade bodies of endothelial cells and the granules of platelets [41]. Within minutes after activation by thrombogenic and inflammatory mediators, P-selectin is mobilized to the plasma membrane to bind neutrophils and monocytes. E-selectin is strongly and rapidly induced on vascular endothelial cells by cytokines such as IL-1β and tumor necrosis factor-α (TNF-α) [42, 43]. All selectins recognize a sialylated carbohydrate determinant on their counterreceptors [44]. E-selectin and P-selectin recognize the tetrasaccharide sialyl Lewis^x and its isomer sialyl Lewis^a [45].

Supporting an important role for leukocyte adhesion by P-selectin and E-selectin after focal cerebral ischemia, several laboratories have recently demonstrated an elevated soluble E-selectin level in the serum of stroke patients and expression of E-selectin and P-selectin in the experimental MCA occlusion. In patients with acute ischemic stroke, the level of soluble E-selectin was significantly elevated at 8 h and persisted up to 24 h and returned to basal levels 72 h after onset of stroke [46]. The transient expression of E-selectin has been mapped in rat brain after focal cerebral ischemia. E-selectin mRNA was detected in the ischemic hemisphere as early as 2 h of reperfusion after transient (2 h) of MCA occlusion and was markedly elevated at 10 h of reperfusion [47, 48]. The elevated E-selectin mRNA persisted up to 22 h, then decreased at 46 h of reperfusion. E-selectin mRNA was no longer detected after 46 h of reperfusion. In permanent MCA occlusion, the level of E-selectin mRNA increased at 6 h, peaked at 12 h and persisted for 48 h after onset of MCA occlusion in rats [49]. The expression of E-selectin mRNA occurred earlier after transient cerebral ischemia than after permanent ischemia. This parallels the more rapid time course of accumulation of neutrophils in transient versus permanent MCA occlusion, and suggests that reperfusion injury is a trigger for rapid transcription of E-selectin mRNA.

E-selectin expression identified by immunohistochemistry is restricted to cerebral microvascular endothelial cells after transient MCA occlusion in the rat [48]. E-selectin immunoreactivity was first observed on microvessels within the ischemic lesion upon reperfusion (fig. 3a) and peaked at 10 and 22 h of reperfusion in ischemic area (fig. 3b, c). E-selectin-immunoreactive vessels decreased after 72 h of reperfusion. Up-regulation of P-selectin occurs on precapillary arterioles and postcapillary venules at 2 h of MCA occlusion and persists up to 24 h of reperfusion after 3 h of MCA occlusion in the baboon [50]. However, it is unclear how long up-regulation of P-selectin would last in this model if the experiment extended after 24 h of reperfusion.

In addition to demonstrating expression of E-selectin and P-selectin, Zhang et al. [48] demonstrated a beneficial effect of a novel sialyl Lewis^x-containing oligosaccharide analog (CY-1503), which blocks both E- and P-selectin function [51]. This sialyl Lewis^x-containing oligosaccharide analog was administered to rats upon reperfusion 2 h after onset of MCA occlusion.

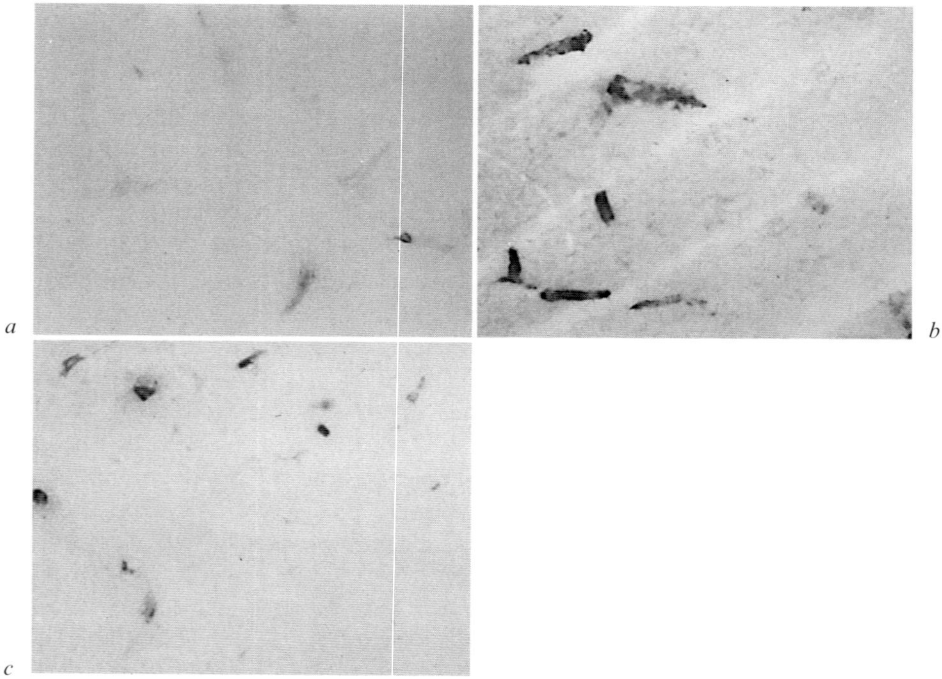

Fig. 3. Photomicrographs of E-selectin-immunoreactive vessels in the ischemic striatum upon reperfusion (*a*), 10 h (*b*) and 22 h of reperfusion after 2 h of MCA occlusion.

Infarct volume and the number of MPO-immunoreactive cells were significantly reduced at 46 h of reperfusion after 2 h of MCA occlusion by treatment with CY-1503 (50 mg/kg).

Soluble L-selectin level in the serum was reduced at day 3 in stroke patients [46]. The decrease of circulating L-selectin suggests that L-selectin may bind to up-regulated endothelial counterreceptors. The effect of inhibition of L-selectin, however, has not been explored in cerebral ischemia and reperfusion injury.

Chemoattractants

For leukocytes to migrate across the vessels and into tissue, a chemotactic gradient is required. Chemoattractants are important in the activation of integrin adhesiveness and in directing the migration of leukocytes [6]. Classical chemoattractants, such as leukotriene B_4 (LTB_4), act broadly on PMNL and monocytes [52]. Chemoattractive cytokines which selectively act on leukocyte subsets are termed chemokines [53]. Chemokines have been divided into two subfamilies by sequence homology and by the sequence around two cysteine residues. The α or cysteine-X-cysteine chemokines tend to act on neutrophils and nonchematopoietic cells, whereas the β or cysteine-cysteine chemokines tend to act on monocytes, eosinophils and lymphocytes. IL-8 belongs to the family of α chemokines [54]. Macrophage inflammatory protein-1 (MIP-1α) and MCP-1 are the members of the β chemokine family [54].

The involvement of classical chemoattractants and chemokines in the ischemic brain has been explored in rats. Increased LTB_4 receptor binding was observed beginning at 12 h and was maximum at 5 days through 15 days in SHR subjected to permanent MCA occlusion [19, 55]. LTB_4 receptor binding following transient (160 min) MCA occlusion increased earlier (6 h of reperfusion) than that following permanent MCA occlusion.

Cytokine-induced neutrophil chemoattractant (CINC) mRNA, a member of the IL-8 family, was significantly induced in the ischemic cortex from 6–24 h with a peak at 12 h after MCA occlusion in SHR [56]. CINC was also present in the ischemic brain after transient (1 h) MCA occlusion in Wistar rat. The CINC/IL-8 level in the ischemic brain was detected at 3 h, peaked at 12 h and reduced at 24–48 h of reperfusion by using a rat CINC enzyme-linked immunosorbent assay kit [57]. The time course of expression of chemokines for monocytes has been studied in permanent and transient MCA occlusion. MCP-1 and MIP-1α mRNA were detected at 6 h, peaked at 24–48 h and attenuated at 96 h after MCA occlusion in Wistar rats [58]. Immunohistochemistry revealed that endothelial cells and macrophage-like cells expressed MCP-1 and activated astrocytes expressed MIP-1α in the ischemic area [58]. The presence of MCP-1 in ischemic brain was confirmed by a study in SHR [59]. A significant increase of expression of MCP-1 mRNA was detected in the ischemic cortex at 12–24 h and remained elevated up to 120 h after MCA occlusion. However, MCP-1 mRNA level significantly increased at 3 h and persisted up to 48 h after transient (160 min) MCA occlusion. These data suggest that ischemic brain produces endogenous chemokines such as IL-8, MCP-1 and MIP-1a which may be responsible for the recruitment of neutrophils and monocytes into the ischemic tissue. Chemokines are likely responsible for activation of microglia after focal cerebral ischemia. In addition, MCP-1 and MIP-1α are not only monocyte chemoattractants but also are major lymphocyte chemoattractants [6, 60]. Therefore, expression of MCP-1 and MIP-1α after focal cerebral ischemia may provide signals required to activate integrin adhesiveness and emigration of both monocytes and lymphocytes into the ischemic tissue. However, in the absence of evidence for inhibition of these chemokines by selective antagonists or antibodies in cerebral ischemia, the role of chemokines in the evolution of inflammatory response to ischemic cell damage after cerebral ischemia remains to be determined.

Integrins

Although selectin-mediated rolling appears to be a prerequisite for leukocyte firm adherence to blood vessels, selectin-dependent adhesion of leukocytes does not lead to firm adhesion and transmigration unless the integrin is engaged [6, 61, 62]. For neutrophils, firm adhesion requires activation of β_2 integrin family, resulting in neutrophil binding to one of the intercellular adhesion molecules located on the surface of endothelial cells.

The leukocyte β_2 integrin family consists of three distinct α chains designated α_L (CD11a), α_M (CD11b), and α_X (CD11c) associated with a common β_2 chain (CD18) [61]. The CD11a/CD18, CD11b/CD18 and CD11c/CD18 integrins are also called lymphocyte function-associated antigen-1 (LFA-1), Mac-1 and p150,95, respectively. The ligands for these integrins are the immunoglobulin superfamily member, ICAM, and fibrinogen, and complement fragments (iC3b) [6, 63].

Up-regulation of CD11a and CD18 has been observed in patients with ischemic stroke and transient ischemic attacks (TIA). Using immunofluorescence phenotyping and flow cytometry, Kim et al. [64] showed that CD11a was significantly increased in patients with stroke and TIA [64]. CD18, however, was increased in patients only with TIA within 72 h after onset of ischemia.

Using monoclonal antibodies (mAb) with the ability to block CD11b and/or CD18 function without causing neutropenia, several groups have examined the role of CD11b and CD18 in cerebral ischemia. The effects of anti-CD11b and anti-CD18 antibodies on a rat model of MCA occlusion have been investigated in a series of experiments by using a mAb directed against rat CD11b epitope (1B6c) and a mAb against rat CD18 epitope (CL26). Both antibodies have been shown to inhibit rat neutrophil adherence to endothelial cells [65, 66]. Intravenous administration of mAb 1B6c or CL26 upon reperfusion after 2 h of MCA occlusion reduced infarct volume as well as MPO activity and improved physiological response when animals were sacrificed at 46 h or 166 h of reperfusion [67, 68]. The beneficial effect of administration of antibody against CD11b on this model has been seen even when mAb 1B6c was administered at 1 or 2 h of reperfusion after 2 h of MCA occlusion [68, 69]. In contrast, no effect was observed on infarct volume and MPO activity in permanent MCA occlusion when mAb 1B6c was given 2 h after MCA occlusion [70]. These data provide evidence that CD11b and CD18 contribute to reperfusion injury and that leukocytes may contribute to ischemic cell damage that occurs after transient (2 h) MCA occlusion in rats. Administration of a mAb against CD18 (IB4) at 15 min before reperfusion increased reflow in microvessels in baboons subjected to 3 h of MCA occlusion and 1 h of reperfusion [32]. However, no beneficial effects on neurological outcome and CBF as well as infarct volume were observed in rabbits and cats treated with mAb against CD18, respectively.

Preadministration of mAb against CD18 in a rabbit model of microsphere cerebral emboli did not improve neurological outcome at 18 h after the insult [12]. This result is not in conflict with the data obtained from rats, since the emboli likely produced a permanent occlusion without reperfusion. Takeshima et al. [71] showed that administration of mAb against CD18 between 40 and 50 min of MCA occlusion did not improve CBF and did not reduce infarct volume as quantified by triphenyltetrazolium chloride (TTC) staining in cats subjected to 90 min of MCA occlusion and 180 min of reperfusion. The failure to find a benefit in this study may be due to using an end point of ischemia at 3 h of reperfusion since the infarct size is not mature at this time.

Matsuo et al. [72] demonstrated a beneficial effect of a mAb against rat CD11a (WT1) administered 15 min before and immediately after reperfusion in rats subjected to 1 h of MCA occlusion and 24 h of reperfusion. Infarct volume, brain edema formation and MPO activity were all significantly reduced at 24 h after reperfusion by the treatment. The efficacy of an anti-CD18 antibody given as an adjunct to thrombolytic therapy to interfere the leukocyte response after ischemia-reperfusion has been assessed. Bowes et al. [73] employed a thrombolytic agent (rt-PA) and anti-CD18 antibody in a rabbit model of multiple cerebral emboli, to test the effects of this combined approach on cerebral ischemia. In this study, animals received 1 mg/kg of anti-CD18 antibody at 5 min after embolization. Three mg/kg of rt-PA was administered at 30 min of postembolization. The neurological impairment of the animals was rated 18 h later. The combined therapy did not enhance the effect of either intervention alone. However, this study did not evaluate whether an adjunctive therapy with rt-PA and anti-CD18 antibody could prolong the therapeutic window for thrombolytic treatment.

The above studies suggest that mAbs direct against β_2 integrin of α chains CD11a, CD11b, and the common β_2 chain CD18 are effective at reducing focal cerebral ischemic reperfusion injury. However, the contribution of CD11c and other integrins such as very late antigen-4 (VLA-4) to ischemic cell damage after MCA occlusion remains to be determined.

Administration of antibodies may cause immunogenicity, and immune complex disease [74]. Instead of treatment with antibodies, other approaches to inhibit CD11b/CD18-mediated ischemia and reperfusion injury are being explored. A recombinant neutrophil inhibitor factor (rNIF), originally found in the hookworm, is a 41-kD glycoprotein ligand of CD11b/CD18 [74, 75]. This protein potently inhibits adhesion of activated human neutrophils to endothelial cells in vitro [76]. The effect of rNIF on cerebral ischemia has been investigated. Rats were subjected to 2 h of MCA occlusion and a bolus of rNIF was administered at the time of reperfusion followed by continuous infusion of rNIF for 48 h [77]. Administration of rNIF to rats reduced the volume of cerebral infarction by more than 48% and reduced the number of neutrophils accumulated in ischemic tissue by 33% as well as significantly improved neurological deficits. Another approach is to employ a peptide to block adhesion molecules. A 20-mer filamentous hemagglutinin peptide containing the Arg-Gly-Asp (RGD) triplet, the cell adhesion motif, decreases ligand binding by CD11b/CD18 [78, 79]. This peptide inhibits neutrophil adherence and transendothelial migration in vitro and impedes recruitment of leukocytes into the cerebrospinal fluid in experimental meningitis in vivo [80]. Administration of this peptide upon reperfusion and at 2, 4, 6, 8, 22, and 30 h of reperfusion after 2 h of MCA occlusion in rats significantly reduced infarct volume (36%) and reduced the number of MPO-immunoreactive cells (38%) [81]. The reduction in infarct volume achieved by this peptide is comparable to that reported for the anti-CD11b or anti-CD18 antibodies. Therefore, a peptide which is potentially less immunogenic than antibodies will likely provide the future direction of therapeutic intervention.

Immunoglobulin Superfamily Members

Several immunoglobulin superfamily members, expressed on endothelium, bind to integrins expressed on leukocytes [6, 82]. Important ligands for the CD11/CD18 integrins are ICAM-1 (CD54) and ICAM-2 [83, 84]. These molecules are constitutively expressed on the endothelial cells. The CD11a/CD18 and CD11b/CD18 integrins bind to ICAM-1 in different regions of the molecule [85–87]. ICAM-1 expression can be augmented by cytokines such as IL-1β and TNF-α or γ-interferon. The up-regulation of ICAM-1 has been observed in acute human ischemic stroke, in human cerebral infarction and in animal models of MCA occlusion. The levels of soluble ICAM-1 in the serum increased in the patients with vascular risk factors and acute ischemic stroke [46]. The transient up-regulation of ICAM-1 identified by immunohistochemistry occurred on endothelium of postcapillary vessels at 1 and 4 h of reperfusion in baboons subjected to 3 h of MCA occlusion [50]. The upregulation of ICAM-1 was not detected at 24 h of reperfusion in this model. In contrast, the persistent up-regulation of ICAM-1 was found in rat models of

MCA occlusion and in photothrombosis. The temporal profiles of ICAM-1 protein and mRNA expression have simultaneously been demonstrated in rat models of the transient and permanent MCA occlusion in two different laboratories.

Significantly elevated ICAM-1 mRNA level in the ischemic cortex was detected at 3 h, peaked at 6–12 h and remained elevated up to 5 days after the permanent coagulated MCA in SHR [88]. The expression of ICAM-1 mRNA level was significantly increased at 1 h of reperfusion, peaked at 12 h and persisted to 5 days of reperfusion after 160 min after MCA occlusion [88]. In a suture model of MCA occlusion in Wistar rats, the expression of ICAM-1 was elevated at 1 h of MCA occlusion, maximized at 10 h of reperfusion after onset of 2 h of MCA occlusion and persisted up to 168 h of reperfusion [89]. ICAM-1 protein significantly increased at 2 h of reperfusion, maximized at 46 h and persisted up to 166 h of reperfusion after 2 h of MCA occlusion [89]. In a long-term (60 days) study of photochemically induced focal ischemia, overexpression of ICAM-1 was observed at 1 day, peaked at 5 and 6 days and lasted for 7 days after photothrombosis [23]. ICAM-1 immunoreactivity was not found after day 14 [23]. The elevated ICAM-1 expression was localized in microvascular endothelial cells in the ischemic lesion in all these studies. The persistent elevated expression of ICAM-1 after focal cerebral ischemia is supported by a postmortem human study [90]. Upregulation of ICAM-1 was observed in microvessels in human cerebral cortical infarct of 4–5 days after stroke.

ICAM-1 provides dynamic 'position-specific' information to guide leukocyte localization during the course of inflammatory response. The finding that MCA occlusion and reperfusion increases ICAM-1 expression suggests that blocking ICAM-1, although not a sufficient event to prevent neutrophil recruitment in ischemic tissue, will likely reduce neutrophil infiltration into the tissue and thereby reduce ischemic cell damage. This hypothesis has been tested by specific studies of the effect of mAb direct against ICAM-1 treatment on infarct size, functional outcome and neutrophil accumulation in different animals of focal cerebral ischemia. Clark et al. [12] and Bowes et al. [91] studied the effect of mAb against ICAM-1 on reducing ischemic injury in rabbit models of multiple brain emboli with or without reperfusion. Treatment with anti-ICAM-1 significantly reduced the number of emboli required to produce neurological impairment at 18 h in rabbits injected with multiple microclot cerebral emboli, whereas no benefit was found with anti-ICAM-1 treatment in the cerebral microsphere emboli model.

The difference between these two models is that autologous blood clots may undergo spontaneous lysis which allows reperfusion when compared to the nondissolvable microspheres. Therefore, these data suggest that anti-ICAM-1 treatment is effective in a reperfusion model, but not a nonreperfusion model. This hypothesis has been supported by work done in our laboratory in a rat suture model of MCA occlusion. We have recently demonstrated that administration of an antibody against ICAM-1 (1A29) at 1 h of reperfusion significantly reduced the infarct volume in rats subjected to 2 h of MCA occlusion and 7 days of reperfusion [92]. In contrast, treatment with anti-ICAM-1 did not reduce infarct volume in rats subjected to 7 days of the permanent MCA occlusion [92]. The finding that delayed (3 h postischemia) treatment with anti-ICAM-1 is beneficial in transient MCA occlusion is consistent with the time of up-regulation of ICAM-1 which occurred at 2 h of reperfusion after 2 h of MCA occlusion. In addition to reducing infarct volume, treatment with anti-ICAM-1 also significantly reduced PMNL infiltration. Rats administered anti-ICAM-1 antibody upon reperfusion after 2 h of MCA occlusion exhibited a 40% reduction in their infarct volume and 50% reduction in the MPO activity [93]. Using the same antibody (1A29), Matsuo et al. [72] also showed that anti-ICAM-1 antibody reduced infarct volume, brain edema and neutrophil accumulation measured by an MPO activity assay in rats subjected to 1 h of MCA occlusion and 24 h of reperfusion. These studies indicate the ability of anti-ICAM-1 treatment to reduce neutrophil infiltration and thereby to reduce ischemic cell damage.

The hypothesis that an anti-ICAM-1 antibody administered as an adjunct to thrombolytic therapy would have a synergistic effect on reperfusion injury has been tested in a rabbit model of multiple cerebral clot emboli. When rt-PA alone was given 2 h after the onset of ischemia there was no benefit in the ischemic rabbits [73]. However, rabbits treated with anti-ICAM-1 at 15 minutes and rt-PA at 2 h after embolization, respectively, showed a significant reduction in neurologic injury.

The above studies suggest that anti-ICAM-1 therapy may be clinically useful in stroke. A double-blind, randomized, placebo-controlled, parallel-group trial of the efficacy and safety of anti-ICAM-1 compared to placebo for treatment of acute ischemic stroke is currently underway.

Summary: The data described above suggest that antiadhesion molecule antibodies reduce accumulation of PMNL in the ischemic brain and thereby reduce ischemic cell damage after transient MCA occlusion. It is, however, important to keep in mind that these antibodies may reduce ischemic cell damage not necessarily by reducing neutrophil migration into ischemic tissue, but by a nonspecific mechanism such as reducing oxidative bursts and protease release from inflammatory cells [94].

Although the above studies have led to a paradigm of selectins, integrins and immunoglobulin superfamily adhesion molecules as critical mediators of inflammatory response after focal cerebral ischemia, additional adhesion molecules that may also play roles in inflammation-mediated cerebral ischemic cell damage remain to be identified.

The temporal profile of expression of adhesion molecules and chemoattractants is generally consistent with the sequence of accumulation of leukocytes in the ischemic brain. Intervention with antibodies and pharmaceutical compounds against adhesion molecules is beneficial after transient MCA occlusion in animals. These findings may lead to clinical applications in stroke therapy. However, there are still many unanswered questions. Although upregulation of IL-1β and TNF-α which appear to play an important role in the induction of adhesion molecules and chemokines have been observed in the ischemic brain in SHR after MCA occlusion, it is not known how these cytokines regulate expression of adhesion molecules and chemokines in cerebral ischemia [95, 96]. Is expression of these genes regulated through the nuclear transcription factor NF-κB after cerebral ischemia? Resolution of these issues may provide novel therapeutic directions in the treatment of cerebral ischemia.

Acknowledgments

The authors thank Denice Janus for her assistance in the preparation of the manuscript. This work was supported by NINDS grants PO1 NS23393, RO1 NS33627 and RO1 NS34184.

References

1 Kochanek PM, Hallenbeck JM, Polymorphonuclear leukocytes and monocytes/macrophages in the pathogenesis of cerebral ischemia and stroke. Stroke 1992;23:1367–1379.

2 Sörnäs R, Östlund H, Müller R: Cerebrospinal fluid cytology after stroke. Arch Neurol 1972;26: 489–501.

3 Garcia JH, Kamijyo Y: Cerebral infarction. Evolution of histopathological changes after occlusion of a middle cerebral artery in primates. J Neuropathol Exp Neurol 1974;33:409–421.

4 Patarroyo M, Prieto J, Rincon J, Timonen T, Lundberg C, Lindbom L, Asjo B, Gahmberg CG: Leukocyte-cell adhesion: A molecular process fundamental in leukocyte physiology. Immunol Rev 1990;114:67–108.

5 Bevilacqua MP: Endothelial-leukocyte adhesion molecules. Annu Rev Immunol 1993;11:767–804.

6 Springer TA: Traffic signals on endothelium for lymphocyte recirculation and leukocyte emigration. Annu Rev Physiol 1995;57:827–872.

7 Butcher EC: Leukocyte-endothelial cell recognition: Three (or more) steps to specificity and diversity. Cell 1991;67:1033–1036.

8 Williams FM, Kus M, Tanda K, Williams TJ: Effect of duration of ischaemia on reduction of myocardial infarct size by inhibition of neutrophil accumulation using an anti-CD18 monoclonal antibody. Br J Pharmacol 1994;111:1122–1128.

9 Jaeschke H, Farhood A, Bautista AP, Spolarics Z, Spitzer JJ, Smith CW: Functional inactivation of neutrophils with a Mac-1 (CD11b/CD18) monoclonal antibody protects against ischemia/reperfusion injury in rat liver. Hepatology 1993;17:15–23.

10 Kelly KJ, Williams WW, Colvin RB, Bonventre JV: Antibody to intercellular adhesion molecule 1 protects the kidney against ischemic injury. Proc Natl Acad Sci USA 1994;91:812–816.
11 Seekamp A, Till GO, Mullligan MS, Paulson JC, Anderson DA, Miyasaka M, Ward PA: Role of selectins in local and remote tissue injury following ischemia and reperfusion. Am J Pathol 1994; 144:592–598.
12 Clark WM, Madden KP, Rothlein R, Zivin JA: Reduction of central nervous system ischemic injury in rabbits using leukocyte adhesion antibody treatment. Stroke 1991;22:877–883.
13 Chopp M, Zhang RL, Jiang N: The role of adhesion molecules in reducing cerebral ischemic cell damage; in Siesjö BK, Wieloch T (eds): Cellular and Molecular Mechanisms of Ischemic Brain Damage. Philadelphia Lippincott-Raven, 1994, vol 71, pp 315–328.
14 Pozzilli C, Lenzi GL, Argentino C, Carolei A, Rasura M, Signore A, Bozzao L, Pozzilli P: Imaging of leukocytic infiltration in human cerebral infarcts. Stroke 1985;16:251–255.
15 Wang P-Y, Kao C-H, Mui M-Y, Wang S-J: Leukocyte infiltration in acute hemispheric ischemic stroke. Stroke 1993;24:236–240.
16 Hallenbeck JM, Dutka AJ, Tanishima T, Kochanek PM, Kumaroo KK, Thompson CB, Obrenovitch TP, Contreras TJ: Polymorphonuclear leukocyte accumulation in brain regions with low blood flow during the early postischemic period. Stroke 1986;17:246–253.
17 del Zoppo GJ, Schmid-Schonbein GW, Mori E, Copeland BR, Chang C-M: Polymorphonuclear leukocytes occlude capillaries following middle cerebral artery occlusion and reperfusion in baboons. Stroke 1991;22:1276–1283.
18 Barone FC, Hillegass LM, Price WJ, White RF, Lee EV, Feuerstein GZ, Sarau HM, Clark RK, Griswold DE: Polymorphonuclear leukocyte infiltration into cerebral focal ischemic tissue: Myeloperoxidase activity assay and histologic verification. J Neurol Res 1991;29:336–345.
19 Barone FC, Hillegass LM, Tzimas MN, Schmidt DB, Foley JJ, White RF, Price WJ, Feuerstein GZ, Clark RK, Griswold DE, Sarau HM: Time-related changes in myeloperoxidase activity and leukotriene B_4 receptor binding reflect leukocyte influx in cerebral focal stroke. Mol Chem Neuropathol 1995;24:13–30.
20 Zhang ZG, Chopp M: Myeloperoxidase immunoreactive cells in ischemic brain after transient middle cerebral artery occlusion in the rat. Neurosci Res Comm 1997;20:85–91.
21 Garcia JH, Liu KF, Yoshida Y, Lian J, Chen S, del Zoppo GJ: Influx of leukocytes and platelets in an evolving brain infarct (Wistar rat). Am J Pathol 1994;144:1–12.
22 Zhang RL, Chopp M, Garcia JH, Chen H: Temporal profile of ischemic tissue damage, neutrophil response, and vascular plugging following permanent and transient (2H) middle cerebral artery occlusion in the rat. J Neurol Sci 1994;125:3–10.
23 Jander S, Kraemer M, Schroeter M, Witte OT, Stoll G: Lymphocytic infiltration and expression of intercellular adhesion molecule-1 in photochemically induced ischemia of the rat cortex. J Cereb Blood Flow Metab 1995;15:42–51.
24 Morioka T, Kalehua AN, Streit WJ: The microglial reaction in the rat dorsal hippocampus following transient forebrain ischemia. J Cereb Blood Flow Metab 1991;11:966–973.
25 Gehrmann J, Bonnekoh P, Miyazawa T, Hossmann K-A, Kreutzberg GW: Immunocytochemical study of an early microglial activation in ischemia. J Cereb Blood Flow Metab 1992;12:257–269.
26 Morioka T, Kalehua AN, Streit WJ: Characterization of microglial reaction after middle cerebral artery occlusion in rat brain. J Comp Neurol 1993;327:123–132.
27 Korematsu K, Goto S, Nagahiro S, Ushio Y: Microglial response to transient focal cerebral ischemia: An immunocytochemical study on the rat cerebral cortex using anti-phosphotyrosine antibody. J Cereb Blood Flow Metab 1994;14:825–830.
28 Suzumura A, Marunouchi T, Yamamoto H: Morphological transformation of microglia in vitro. Brain Res 1991;545:301–306.
29 Giulian D: Ameboid microglia as effectors of inflammation in the central nervous system. J Neurosci Res 1987;18:155–171.
30 Giulian D, Baker TJ, Shish LN, Lachman LB: Interleukin-1 of the central nervous system is produced by ameboid microglia. J Exp Med 1986;164:594–604.
31 Zhang ZG, Chopp M: Temporal profile of microglial response following transient (2 h) middle cerebral artery occlusion. Brain Res 1997;744:189–198.

32 Mori E, del Zoppo, GJ, Chambers D, Copeland BR, Arfors KE: Inhibition of polymorphonuclear leukocyte adherence suppresses no-reflow after focal cerebral ischemia in baboons. Stroke 1992;23: 712–718.

33 Matsuo Y, Kihara T, Ikeda M, Ninomiya M, Onodera H, Kogure K: Role of neutrophils in radical production during ischemia and reperfusion of the rat brain: Effect of neutrophil depletion on extracellular ascorbyl radical formation. J Cereb Blood Flow Metab 1995;15:941–947.

34 Dutka AJ, Kochanek PM, Hallenbeck JM: Influence of granulocytopenia on canine cerebral ischemia induced by air embolism. Stroke 1989;20:390–395.

35 Bednar MM, Raymond S, McAuliffe T, Lodge PA, Gross CE: The role of neutrophils and platelets in a rabbit model of thromboembolic stroke. Stroke 1991;22:44–50.

36 Chen H, Chopp M, Bodzin G: Neutropenia reduces the volume of cerebral infarct after transient middle cerebral artery occlusion in the rat. Neurosci Res Commun 1992;11:93–99.

37 Matsuo Y, Onodera H, Siga Y, Nakamura M, Ninomiya M, Kihara T, Kogure K: Correlation between myeloperoxidase-quantified neutrophil accumulation and ischemic brain injury in the rat: Effects of neutrophil depletion. Stroke 1994;25:1469–1475.

38 Lasky LA: Selectins: Interpreters of cell-specific carbohydrate information during inflammation. Science 1992;258:964–969.

39 Seekamp A, Till GO, Mullligan MS, Paulson JC, Anderson DA, Miyasaka M, Ward PA: Role of selectins in local and remote tissue injury following ischemia and reperfusion. Am J Pathol 1994; 144:592–598.

40 von Andrian UH, Chambers JD, Berg EL, Michie SA, Karolak D, Ramezani L, Berger EM, Arfors KE, Butcher EC: L-selectin mediates neutrophil rolling in inflamed venules through sialyl Lewis^x-dependent and independent recognition pathways. Blood 1993;82:182–191.

41 McEver RP, Beckstead JH, Moore KL, Marshall-Carlson L, Bainton DF: GMP–140, a platelet alpha-granule membrane protein, is also synthesized by vascular endothelial cells and is localized in Weibel-Palade bodies. J Clin Invest 1989;84:92–99.

42 Bevilacqua MP, Stengelin S, Gimbrone MA Jr, Seed B: Endothelial leukocyte adhesion molecule 1: An inducible receptor for neutrophils related to complement regulatory proteins and lectins. Science 1989;243:1160–1165.

43 Altavilla D, Francesco S, Patrizia C, Mariapatrizia I, Giuseppe MC, Giovanni S, Antonino S, Achille PC: Tumor necrosis factor induces E-selectin production in splanchnic artery occlusion shock. Am J Physiol 1995;268:H1412–H1417.

44 Fukuda J, Spoonce E, Oates JE, Dell A, Klock JC: Structure of sialylated fucosylated lactosaminoglycan isolated from human granulocytes. J Biol Chem 1984;259:10925–10935.

45 Phillips ML, Nudelman E, Gaea FCA, Peter M, Singaal AK, Hakomori S, Paulson JC: ELAM-1 mediates cell adhesion by recognition of a carbohydrate ligand sialyl-Le^x. Science 1990;250: 1130–1132.

46 Fassbender K, Mössner R, Motsch L, Kischka U, Grau A, Hennerici M: Circulating selectin- and immunoglobulin-type adhesion molecules in acute ischemic stroke. Stroke 1995;26:1361–1364.

47 Zhang RL, Chopp M, Zhang ZG, Gautam SC, Anderson DC, Manning AM: Induction of E-selectin mRNA in the brain after transient focal cerebral ischemia in rat (abstract). J Cereb Blood Flow Metab 1995;15:S113.

48 Zhang RL, Chopp M, Zhang ZG, Phillips ML, Rosenbloom CL, Cruz R, Manning A: E-selectin in focal cerebral ischemia and reperfusion in the rat. J Cereb Blood Flow Metab 1996;16:1126–1136.

49 Wang XK, Yue TL, Barone FC, Feuerstein GZ: Demonstration of increased endothelial-leukocyte adhesion molecule-1 mRNA expresssion in rat ischemic cortex. Stroke 1995;26:1665–1669.

50 Okada Y, Copeland BR, Mori E, Tung M-M, Thoms WS, del Zoppo GJ: P-selectin and intercellular adhesion molecule-1 expression after brain ischemia reperfusion. Stroke 1994;25:202–211.

51 Lefer DL, Flynn DM, Phillips L, Ratcliffe M, Buda AJ: A novel sialyl Lewis^x analog attenuates neutrophil accumulation and myocardial necrosis after ischemia and reperfusion. Circulation 1994; 90:2390–2401.

52 Snyderman R, Uhing RJ: Chemoattractant stimulus-response coupling, in Gallin JI, Goldstein IM, Snyderman R (eds): Inflammation: Basic Principles and Clinical Correlates. New York, Raven Press, 1992, pp 421–439.

53 Miller MD, Krangel MS: Biology and biochemistry of chemokines: A family of chemotactic and inflammatory cytokines. Crit Rev Immunol 1992;12:17–46.
54 Baggiolini M, Dewald B, Moser B: Interleukin-8 and related chemotactic cytokines – CXC and CC chemokines. Adv Immunol 1994;55:97–179.
55 Barone FC, Schmidt DB, Hillegass LM, Price WJ, White RF, Feuerstein GZ, Clark RK, Lee EV, Griswold DE, Sarau HM: Reperfusion increases neutrophils and leukotriene B_4 receptor binding in rat focal ischemia. Stroke 1992;23:1337–1348.
56 Liu T, Young PR, McDonnell PC, White RF, Barone FC, Feuerstein GZ: Cytokine-induced neutrophil chemoattractant mRNA expressed in cerebral ischemia. Neurosci Lett 1993;164:125–128.
57 Yamasaki Y, Matsue Y, Matsuura N, Onodera H, Itoyama Y, Kogure K: Transient increase of cytokine-induced neutrophil chemoattractant, a member of the interleukin-8 family, in ischemic brain areas after focal ischemia in rats. Stroke 1995;26:318–323.
58 Kim JS, Gautam SC, Chopp M, Zaloga C, Jones ML, Ward PA, Welch KMA: Expression of monocyte chemoattractant protein-1 and macrophage inflammatory protein-1α after focal cerebral ischemia in rat. J Neuroimmunol 1995;56:127–134.
59 Wang X, Yue T-L, Barone FC, Feuerstein GZ: Monocyte chemoattractant protein-1 messenger RNA expression in rat ischemic cortex. Stroke 1995;26:661–666.
60 Carr MW, Roth SJ, Luther E, Rose SS, Springer TA: Monocyte chemoattractant protein-1 is a major T lymphocyte chemoattractant. Proc Natl Acad Sci USA 1994;91:3652–3656.
61 Kishimoto TK, Larson RS, Corbi AL, Dustin ML, Staunton DE, Springer TA: The leukocyte integrins. Adv Immunol 1989;46:149–182.
62 Lawrence MB, Springer TA: Leukocytes roll on a selectin at physiological flow rates: Distinction from and prerequisite for adhesion through integrins. Cell 1991;65:859–873.
63 Argenbright LW, Barton RW: Interactions of leukocyte integrins with intercellular adhesion molecule 1 in the production of inflammatory vascular injury in vivo. J Clin Invest 1992;89:259–272.
64 Kim JS, Chopp M, Chen H, Levine SR, Carey JL, Welch KMA: Adhesive glycoproteins CD11a and CD18 are upregulated in the leukocytes from patients with ischemic stroke and TIA. J Neurol Sci 1995;18:634–637.
65 Mulligan MS, Varani J, Warren JS, Till GO, Smith CW, Anderson DC, Todd RF III, Ward PA: Role of beta-2 integrins of rat neutrophils in complement- and oxygen radical-mediated acute inflammatory injury. J Immunol 1992;149:1847–1857.
66 Mulligan MS, Wilson GP, Todd RF III, Rusche JR, Smith CW, Anderson DC, Varani J, Issekutz T, Miyasaka M, Tamatani T, Ward PA: Role of B_1, B_2 integrins and ICAM-1 in lung injury following deposition of IgG and IgA immune complexes. J Immunol 1993;150:2407–2417.
67 Chen H, Chopp M, Zhang RL, Bodzin G, Chen Q, Rusche JR, Todd RJ III: Anti-CD11b monoclonal antibody reduces ischemic cell damage after transient focal cerebral ischemia in rat. Ann Neurol 1994;35:447–452.
68 Zhang ZG, Chopp M, Tang WX, Jiang N, Zhang RL: Postischemic treatment (2–4 h) with anti-CD11b and anti-CD18 monoclonal antibodies are neuroprotective after transient (2 h) focal cerebral ischemia in the rat. Brain Res 1995;698:79–85.
69 Chopp M, Zhang R-L, Chen H, Li Y, Jiang N, Rusche JR: Post-ischemic administration of an anti-Mac-1 antibody reduces ischemic cell damage after transient middle cerebral artery occlusion in the rat. Stroke 1994;25:869–876.
70 Jiang N, Zhang RL, Chen H, Chopp M: Anti-CD11b monoclonal antibody reduces ischemic cell damage after transient (2 h) but not after permanent MCA occlusion in the rat. Neurosci Res Commun 1994;15:85–93.
71 Takeshima R, Kirsch JR, Koehler RC, Gomoll AW, Traystman RJ: Monoclonal leukocyte antibody does not decrease in injury of transient focal cerebral ischemia in cats. Stroke 1992;23:247–252.
72 Matsuo Y, Onodera H, Shiga Y, Shozuhara H, Ninomiya M, Kihara T, Tamatani T, Miyasaka M, Kogure K: Role of cell adhesion molecules in brain injury after transient middle cerebral artery occlusion in the rat. Brain Res 1994;656:344–352.
73 Bowes MP, Rothlein R, Fagan SC, Zivin JA: Monoclonal antibodies preventing leukocyte activation reduce experimental neurologic injury and enhance efficacy of thrombolytic therapy. Neurology 1995;45:815–819.

74 Ward PA, Mulligan MS: Strategies for in vivo blocking of adhesion molecules. New Drugs Allergy Asthma 1993;43:173–186.
75 Moyle M, Foster DL, McGrath DE, Brown SM, Laroche Y, De Meutter J, Stanssens P, Bogowitz CA, Fried VA, Ely JA, Soule HR, Vlasuk GP: A hookworm glycoprotein that inhibits neutrophil function is a ligand of the integrin CD11b/CD18. J Biol Chem 1994;269:10008–10015.
76 Muchowski PJ, Zhang L, Chang ER, Soule HR, Plow EF, Moyle M: Functional interaction between the integrin antagonist neutrophil inhibitory factor and the I domain of CD11b/CD18. J Biol Chem 1994;269:26419–26423.
77 Jiang N, Moyle M, Soule HR, Rote WE, Chopp M: Neutrophil inhibitory factor is neuroprotective after focal ischemia in rats. Ann Neurol 1995;38:935–942.
78 Relman D, Tuomanen E, Falkow S, Golenbock DT, Saukkonen K, Wright SD: Recognition of a bacterial adhesion by an integrin: Macrophage CRS α_M β_2, CD11b/CD18, binds filamentous hemagglutinin of *Bordetella pertussis*. Cell 1990;61:1375–1382.
79 Saukkonen K, Cabellos C, Burroughs M, Prasad S, Tuomanen E: The role of the interaction between *Bordetella pertussis* and macrophage integrin CR3 in pulmonary colonization. J Exp Med 1991; 173:1143–1149.
80 Rozdzinski E, Spellerberg B, van der Flier M, Bhattacharyya C, Hoepelman AI, Moran MA, Jarpe A, Putney SD, Starzyk RM, Tuomanen E: Peptide from a prokaryotic adhesin blocks leukocyte migration in vitro and in vivo. J Infect Dis 1995;172:785–793.
81 Zhang RL, Chopp M, Tang WX, Zhang ZG, Putney SD, Starzyk RM: Synthetic peptide derived from the *Bordetella pertussis* bacterium reduces infarct volume after transient middle cerebral artery occlusion in the rat. Neurology 1996;46:1437–1441.
82 Rothlein R, Czajkowski M, Kishimoto TK: Intercellular adhesion molecule-1 in the inflammatory response; in Hogg N (ed): Integrins and ICAM-1 in Immune Responses. Chem Immunol. Basel, Karger, 1991, vol 50, pp 135–142.
83 Diamond MS, Staunton DE, Marlin SD, Springer TA: Binding of the integrin Mac-1 (CD11b/CD18) to the third Ig-like domain of ICAM-1 (CD54) and its regulation by glycosylation. Cell 1991;65:961–971.
84 deFougerolles AR, Qin X, Springer TA: Characterization of the function of ICAM-3 and comparison to ICAM-1 and ICAM-2 in immune responses. J Exp Med 1994;179:619–629.
85 Smith CW, Marlin SD, Rothlein R, Toman C, Anderson DC: Cooperative interaction of LFA-1 and Mac-1 with intercellular adhesion molecule-1 in facilitating adherence and transendothelial migration of human neutrophils in vitro. J Clin Invest 1989;83:2008–2017.
86 Lo SK, van Seventer GA, Levin SM, Wright SD: Two leukocyte receptors (CD11a/CD18 and CD11b/CD18) mediate transient adhesion to endothelium by binding to differenct ligands. J Immunol 1989; 143:3325–3329.
87 Luscinskas FW, Cybulsky MI, Kiely JM, Peckins CS, Davis VM, Gimbrone MA Jr: Cytokine-activated human endothelial monolayers support enhanced neutrophil transmigration via a mechanism involving both endothelial-leukocyte adhesion molecule-1 and intercellular adhesion molecule-1. J Immunol 1991;146: 1617.
88 Wang X, Siren A-L, Liu Y, Yue T-L, Barone FC, Feuerstein GZ: Upregulation of intercellular adhesion molecule 1 (ICAM-1) on brain microvascular endothelial cells in rat ischemic cortex. Mol Brain Res 1994;26:61–68.
89 Zhang RL, Chopp M, Zaloga C, Zhang ZG, Jiang N, Gautam SC, Tang WX, Tsang W, Anderson DC, Manning AM: The temporal profiles of ICAM-1 protein and mRNA expression after transient MCA occlusion in the rat. Brain Res 1995;682:182–188.
90 Sobel RRA, Mitchell ME, Fondren G: Intercellular adhesion molecule-1 (ICAM-1) in cellular immune reactions in the human central nervous system. Am J Pathol 1990;136:1309–1316.
91 Bowes MP, Zivin JA, Rothlein R: Monoclonal antibody to the ICAM-1 adhesion site reduces neurological damage in a rabbit cerebral embolism stroke model. Exp Neurol 1993;119:215–219.
92 Zhang RL, Chopp M, Jiang N, Tang WX, Prostak J, Manning AM: Anti-ICAM-1 antibody reduces ischemic cell damage after transient but not permanent MCA occlusion in the Wistar rat. Stroke 1995;26:1438–1443.

93 Zhang RL, Chopp M, Li Y, Zaloga C, Jiang N, Jones M, Miyasaka M, Ward P: Anti-ICAM-1 antibody reduces ischemic cell damage after transient middle cerebral artery occlusion in the rat. Neurology 1994;44:1747–1751.

94 Hill J, Lindsay T, Rusche J, Valeri CR, Shepro D, Hechtman HB: A Mac-1 antibody reduces liver and lung injury but not neutrophil sequestration after intestinal ischemia-reperfusion. Surgery 1992; 112:166–172.

95 Liu T, Mcdonnell PC, Young PR, White RF, Siren AL, Hallenbeck JM, Barone FC, Feuerstein GZ: Interleukin-1β mRNA expression in ischemic rat cortex. Stroke 1993;24:1746–1751.

96 Liu T, Clark RK, McDonnell PC, Young PR, White RF, Barone FC, Feuerstein GZ: Tumor necrosis factor-α expression in ischemic neurons. Stroke 1994;25:1481–1488.

Michael Chopp, PhD, Henry Ford Hospital, Neurology Department, 2799 West Grand Boulevard, Detroit, MI 48202 (USA)

Hsu CY (ed): Ischemic Stroke: From Basic Mechanisms to New Drug Development.
Monogr Clin Neurosci. Basel, Karger, 1998, vol 16, pp 65–88

Temperature Influences on Ischemic Brain Injury[1]

Myron D. Ginsberg

Cerebral Vascular Disease Research Center, Department of Neurology,
University of Miami School of Medicine, Miami, Fla., USA

Historical Background

The therapeutic applications of hypothermia have a venerable if uneven history. Hypothermia was first applied to induce analgesia for surgical procedures such as limb amputation. In the early decades of this century, local and generalized cooling were variously used to treat malignancies [1], head injury [2], and other conditions, in the course of which clinical observations were recorded [3]: retrograde amnesia was described at temperatures below 34 °C, dysarthria at 34 °C, aphasia at 27 °C and loss of the pupillary light reflex at 26 °C. Sudden cardiac failure, presumably due to ventricular fibrillation, occurred commonly. During World War II, the Nazis conducted brutal human hypothermia experimentation on concentration camp victims – atrocities which were brought to light at the Nuremberg trials [4].

The concept of hypothermia-induced organ protection was applied to cardiac surgical procedures requiring circulatory interruption, in which there was thus a risk of cerebral ischemia. Efforts to define safe durations of hypothermic circulatory arrest led to its eventual application in the operative setting of pump oxygenation and extracorporeal cooling [5] – a technique routinely employed today in patients undergoing cardiac surgery. Hypothermia was also applied during neurosurgical procedures, particularly during the clipping of cerebral aneurysms [6] and removal of arteriovenous malformations – procedures typically necessitating vascular occlusion or controlled hypotension. Today, these applications are generally confined to difficult cases; in such

[1] Our studies are supported by USPHS Grant NS 05820.

instances, pump oxygenation and cardiac bypass at temperatures as low as 4–15 °C have been used [7]. Because profound degrees of intraoperative hypothermia were often complicated by ventricular fibrillation, acidosis, shivering, bleeding dyscrasias and ischemic sensory neuropathies, these hypothermic techniques came to be supplanted by improved neuroanesthetic techniques. Therapeutic hypothermia was applied in the clinic, with variable degrees of success, to treat spontaneous intracerebral hemorrhage, to reduce brain injury following cardiac arrest, and to protect the spinal cord from ischemia following spinal cord injury and during operative aortic occlusion [8]. These studies are reviewed in Ginsberg et al. [9].

In canine studies, it was established that, for each degree decrement in body temperature between 35 and 25 °C, cerebral blood flow decreased by approximately 7%, and oxygen consumption declined correspondingly [10]; brain volume and cerebrospinal fluid pressure also decreased [11]. A 50% reduction in cerebral metabolic rate was documented with hypothermia of 30 °C [12]. Later studies in anesthetized rats confirmed that cerebral oxygen utilization declined linearly over the range of 37–22 °C, and was 65% of normal at temperatures of 30 °C [13]. Profound hypothermia (to 24–25 °C) was shown to be protective in canine models of middle cerebral artery (MCA) occlusion [14, 15] and cerebral contusion [16].

Early efforts to achieve *selective* brain cooling included cold carotid artery perfusion [17], which was applied during intracranial surgery and for open-heart surgery. Mortality and morbidity, however, were very high. Other methods included cerebroventricular perfusion with hypothermic solutions [18]. Experimental studies in monkeys explored cooling of the brain to 14–15 °C by means of a femoral-carotid arterial shunt during 45 min of complete cerebral circulatory arrest; treated animals recovered without a behavioral deficit [19].

Hypothermic Neuroprotection in Global Cerebral Ischemia

A new era in hypothermic neuroprotection was ushered in by experimental observations providing persuasive evidence that even small decrements in brain temperature are able to protect against ischemic brain injury.

Intraischemic Hypothermia

Pioneering observations in rabbits with complete brain ischemia established that the duration of tolerable ischemia compatible with complete functional and pathological recovery could be extended in a continuous fashion from 8–10 min (at 37 °C) up to 40 min when temperature was reduced to 25 °C

[20]. Other experimental hypoxia-ischemia studies supported the notion of metabolic protection with only moderate temperature reductions [21], in some cases as little as 1–3 °C [22]. Despite these indications that the sequelae of ischemia depended sensitively upon temperature, most experimental studies of hypoxia-ischemia carried out before the mid-1980s did not monitor or control the temperature of the ischemic brain but rather considered it sufficient to control rectal temperature alone. In retrospect, this failure contributed to the vexatious variability in the outcome of ostensibly 'standardized' ischemia models [e.g., 23].

In our laboratory, we serendipitiously noted, in the course of a global ischemia study [24], that rats whose scalp tissues were reflected for EEG monitoring showed less ischemic neuropathology than comparably insulted animals with intact scalps. This led to a controlled study to monitor brain temperature directly and to control it independently of rectal temperature, so as to ascsertain whether ischemic neuropathology could be modulated by small brain-temperature differences [25, 26]. In these studies, Wistar rats received 20-min of four-vessel occlusion [27], with reduction of mean arterial blood pressure to 80 mm Hg by blood withdrawal [25]. Despite thermostatic control of rectal temperature at 37 °C by body heating, global forebrain ischemia caused the *brain* temperature to decline initially by approximately 0.5 °C/min, but with considerable inter-animal variability [25]. A controlled study was then carried out, in which brain temperature (as measured by an intrastriatal probe) was intentionally thermostated (via a warming lamp over the head) at either 33, 34, 36, or 39 °C *during* the ischemic insult, but was held at 36 °C before and after the insult in all groups [25]. Histopathology following a 3-day survival revealed, in the 36 °C group, prominent ischemic cell change (ICC) in dorsolateral and central striatum and marked loss of pyramidal neurons in the CA1 sector of hippocampus. By contrast, intraischemic cooling to even 33–34 °C resulted in marked reductions in ICC in both hippocampus (fig. 1) and striatum, which was even more pronounced in the 30 °C group [25]. This study established that as small a decrement as 2 °C in intraischemic brain temperature is neuroprotective, and that core body temperature measurements during ischemia are unreliable indices of *brain* temperature, which must therefore be independently estimated and controlled. Temporalis muscle temperature proved to correlate highly with brain temperature and could be used to estimate it, provided that a calibration curve was constructed under the specific conditions of each experiment.

Other laboratories have fully confirmed neuroprotection by mild intraischemic hypothermia. Thus, in rats with 20 min of 'two-vessel occlusion' (bilateral carotid artery occlusions plus hypotension), in which rectal and skull temperatures were set at levels between 33 and 38 °C, neuronal necrosis following 7-

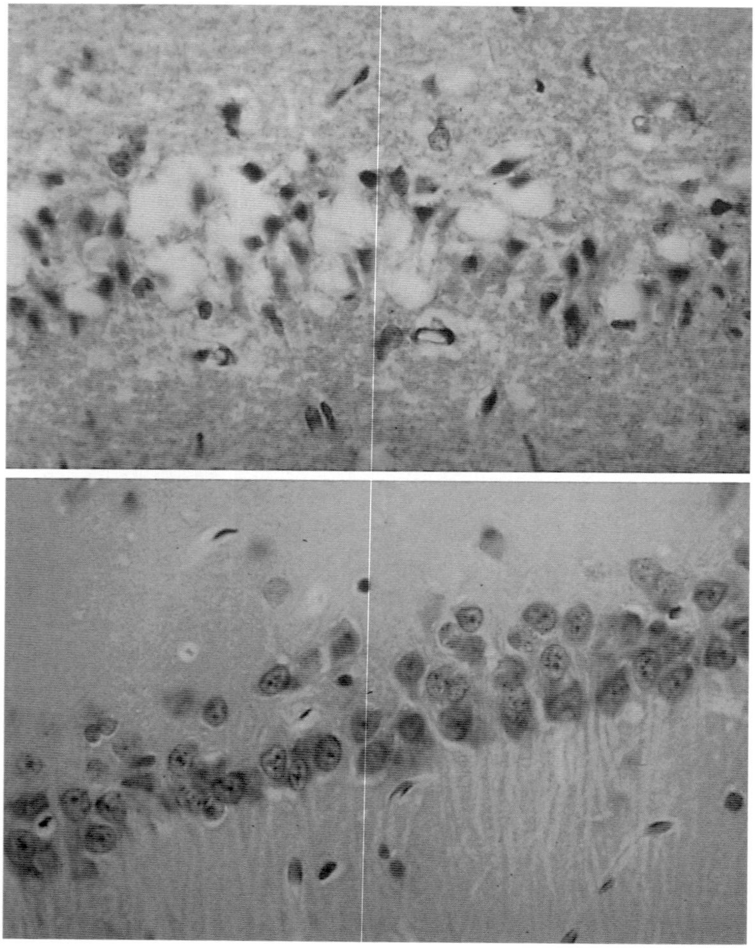

Fig. 1. Hematoxylin- and eosin-stained sections of perfusion-fixed brains 3 days following 20 min global forebrain ischemia. *a* Intraischemic brain temperature 36 °C; pyramidal neurons of hippocampal sector CA1 are completely necrotic. *b* Intraischemic brain temperature 30 °C: CA1 pyramidal neurons are well preserved. ×400.

day survival showed a marked temperature dependence, particularly in the caudoputamen, where severe changes occurred in the 37–38 °C groups but were nearly absent in the 33 and 35 °C groups; in hippocampus; and in neocortex, where a continuous protective trend was evident over the range 38–33 °C [28]. In further studies, this group used whole-body hypothermia of 35 °C (temperature-controlled box with high ambient humidity) [29] with periods of forebrain ischemia of 5, 10, or 15 min. The subicular and CA1 regions of hippocampus were injured by each duration of normothermic ischemia, and in each case protection was seen in the 35 °C groups [30]. Other laboratories have confirmed that even the spontaneous decline of brain temperature which occurs during temperature-*un*controlled ischemic insults [28, 31] confers hippocampal protection when compared to brains held at preischemic (normothermic) levels [32]. Hyperglycemia exacerbates the sequelae of global ischemia, and moderate hypothermia (32–33 °C) under these circumstances increases survival, abolishes postischemic seizures, and diminishes the extent of pathologic changes [33].

A variety of recent moderate-hypothermia studies in larger species – in particular, the work of Safar's group in canine cardiac arrest models – has tended to bear out the major findings of small-animal work. Thus, mild systemic cooling (34 °C) during recirculation and for 1 h after a 12.5-min period of normothermic cardiac arrest improved overall neurologic performance and lowered histopathologic damage scores [34]. These findings wre confirmed in a second study in dogs cooled for 1 h postarrest to 30 or 34 °C, but the use of deep hypothermia (15 °C) worsened cerebral outcome [35]. Delaying the initiation of cooling by 15 min after reperfusion negated the beneficial effect of mild resuscitative hypothermia [36]. In a canine model of complete cerebral ischemia for 12.5 min by arterial hypotension plus intracranial hypertension, it has been recently shown that even a 1–2 °C change in temperature (i.e., 37 vs. 38 vs. 39 °C) significantly alters neurologic outcome and histopathology [37].

Biochemical and Physiologic Correlates of Hypothermic Neuroprotection in Global Ischemia

In our initial studies, we confirmed that intraischemic hypothermic neuroprotection was not attributable to differential decrements in cerebral blood flow (CBF) during ischemia (cortical and striatal CBF were 0.01–0.05 ml/g/min in all temperature groups); likewise, energy metabolite depletion following 20 min ischemia was virtually complete in all groups [25, 38]. (Other studies, however, provide evidence that hypothermia somewhat *delays* the onset of energy metabolite depletion in gerbil forebrain ischemia (32.5 vs. 37.5 °C) [39] and in the postdecapitation canine brain (30 vs. 37 °C) [40]). That a regionally selective pattern of pathologic injury following global ischemia arises despite (eventually) uniform degrees of ATP depletion [39], however, argues against the pathophysiologic importance of differential initial rates of energy metabolite depletion. In a canine model of 10 min cardiac arrest, cerebral lactate accumulation did not differ in hypothermic (33 °C) and normothermic animals [41], whereas another study, employing magnetic resonance spectroscopy during global ischemia in cats, found diminished acidosis and better adenylate recovery in hypothermic (27–34 °C) animals [42].

An extensive study of regional brain energy metabolites in rats with 20 min forebrain ischemia at cranial temperatures of either 30, 37, or 39 °C showed a high degree of striatal, hippocampal and neocortical energy-metabolite recovery (studied at 30 min to 4 h) in all temperature groups, although this was somewhat less complete in the 39 °C groups [43]. Brain free fatty acid (FFA) levels increased following cerebral ischemia; puzzlingly, increases in striatal free stearic and arachidonic levels were higher following ischemia at 30 °C than at 36 °C [38]. As FFA release in ischemia reflects breakdown of phospholipids and/or defective FFA reacylation, these observations seem paradoxical vis-à-vis hypothermic neuroprotection and remain to be satisfactorily explained.

Mild intraischemic hypothermia improves local glucose utilization (lCMRgl) and blood flow measured in the early postischemic period [44] – compatible with improved functional restitution. The brain's capacity for stimulus-induced metabolic activation (as measured by deoxyglucose autoradiography during vibrissae stimulation 1 day following 10 min global ischemia at temperatures of 37 or 30 °C) was also studied. Rats with normothermic ischemia had depressed resting levels of lCMRgl and markedly impaired somotosensory cortical activation, whereas rats with hypothermic ischemia had near-normal resting lCMRgl and preserved activation responses [45]. Correspondingly, postischemic water maze performance was improved by intraischemic hypothermia [46].

Radioisotopic studies of regional cerebral protein synthesis suggest that the protective effect of intraischemic hypothermia (30 °C) on ischemic hippocampal CA1 injury may be mediated by a reversal of the (otherwise expected) postischemic global inhibition of protein synthesis [47].

Specific Cellular Mechanisms of Hypothermic Neuroprotection

Release of Neurotransmitters

Many neurotransmitters and neuromodulators are released into the brain's extracellular space during ischemia [48, 49]. The synthesis, release and uptake of neurotransmitters may be inhibited at decreased temperature [50, 51]. We have shown that the release of the excitatory transmitter glutamate, studied by microdialysis, is markedly depressed by even mild degrees of intraischemic hypothermia: the 7-fold increases in extracellular striatal glutamate levels achieved during 20 min global ischemia are completely blunted by lowering brain temperature to 33 or 30 °C (fig. 2), and the release of dopamine (normally up to 500-fold over resting levels) is blunted by approximately 60% [38, 49, 52]. Others have confirmed the attenuation of ischemia-induced glutamate release at brain temperatures of 31–35 °C [53], and marked attenuation of

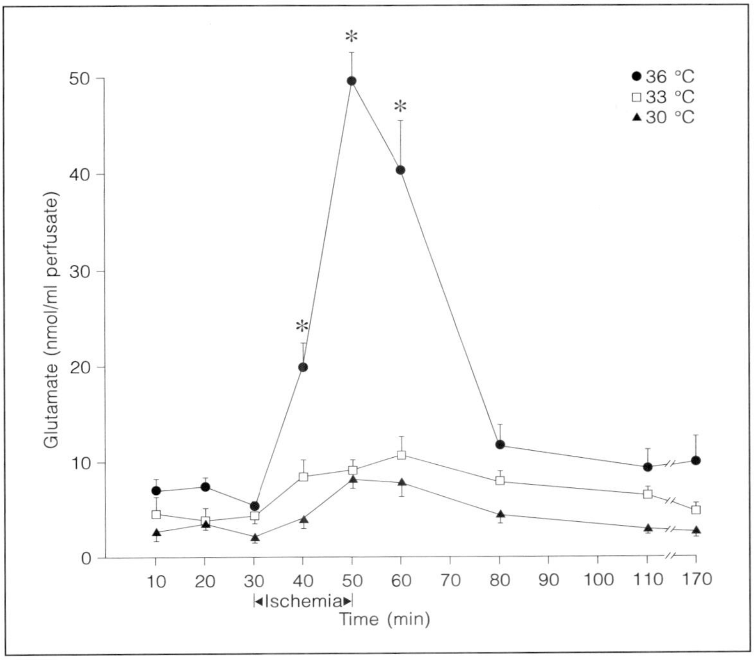

Fig. 2. Microdialysis perfusate levels of glutamate in rats receiving 20 min of global ischemia, whose intraischemic brain temperature was maintained at either 36, 33, or 30 °C. Values represent means ± SEM. In hypothermic rats, the ischemic-induced increase in extracellular glutamate is completely suppressed. * Significantly higher than control values ($p < 0.01$, two-way ANOVA). (Reproduced from Busto et al. [38] with permission.)

glutamate, aspartate, and glycine levels at 20 °C [54]. It is to be noted that extracellular concentrations of glutamate attained during normothermic ischemia [52] are similar to those associated with neurotoxicity in in vitro systems [55]. Many studies have convincingly implicated glutamate-associated excitotoxicity in the pathogenesis of ischemic brain injury [56–58], and dopamine release likewise plays a role in ischemic striatal injury [52, 59]. Thus, the blunting of neurotransmitter release effected by intraischemic hypothermia may be central to its neuroprotective action.

The so-called excitotoxic index (EI), defined as [glutamate] × [glycine]/[GABA], reflects a composite of excitatory (glutamate, glycine) and inhibitory (GABA) neurotransmitter balance [60, 61]. Normothermic rats with 12.5 min global ischemia showed increases in the striatal EI of 7- to 12-fold during early recirculation, whereas postischemic hypothermia (30 °C × 3 h) suppressed this response [62].

Free Radical Activity

The use of intracerebral microdialysis to measure local cerebral production of the adducts 2,3- and 2,5-dihydrobenzoic acid (DHBA) in response to salicylate administration – a fingerprint of hydroxyl radical production – has substantiated the production of free radicals in the course of both global [63, 64] and focal [65] ischemia and fluid-percussion brain injury [66]. Hypothermia (30 °C) during 15 or 20 min global ischemia almost completely suppresses this hydroxyl radical signal (fig. 3) [63, 64], and a similar phenomenon has been observed with post*traumatic* hypothermia [66]. Furthermore, the brain's reduction of its endogenous antioxidants (ascorbate and glutathione) after 3 h transient focal ischemia is lessened by intraischemic hypothermia (33 °C) in rats [67]. In the normothermic focally ischemic rat cortex, hypothermia (33 °C) also abolishes the increase in nitric oxide synthase activity and suppresses cyclic guanosine monophosphate (cGMP) production – two markers of the synthesis of the free radical, nitric oxide (NO) [68]. These data support the suppression of free radical activity as at least one mechanism of hypothermic neuroprotection.

Intracellular Mediators

Calcium/calmodulin-dependent protein kinase II (CaM kinase II), an enzyme responsible for transducing intracellular calcium signals and regulating a variety of cellular processes involving protein phosphorylation [69], is permanently inactivated by brief forebrain ischemia [70], but this can be averted by moderate hypothermia (32 °C) and markedly exacerbated by hyperthermia [71]. The inactivation of this enzyme is thought to be due to a posttranslational modification.

Protein kinase C (PKC) is an important calcium-dependent enzyme activated by inositol phospholipid hydrolysis to diacylglycerol, which is thought to regulate neurotransmitter release and gene expression [72]. Translation of PKC from cytosol to cell membrane and inhibition of the enzyme have been demonstrated in ischemia [73]. Striatal homogenates of rats with hypothermia (27 °C) during 20 min of ischemia, in contrast to normothermic rats, showed no translocation or inhibition [74]. This could be due to a hypothermia-induced cell membrane modification. A recent study from our laboratory has confirmed a significant temperature effect for both membrane-bound and cytosolic PKC, with normothermic-ischemic rats showing sustained (24 h) postischemic depressions in PKC activity, whereas this was not observed following 30 °C ischemia [75].

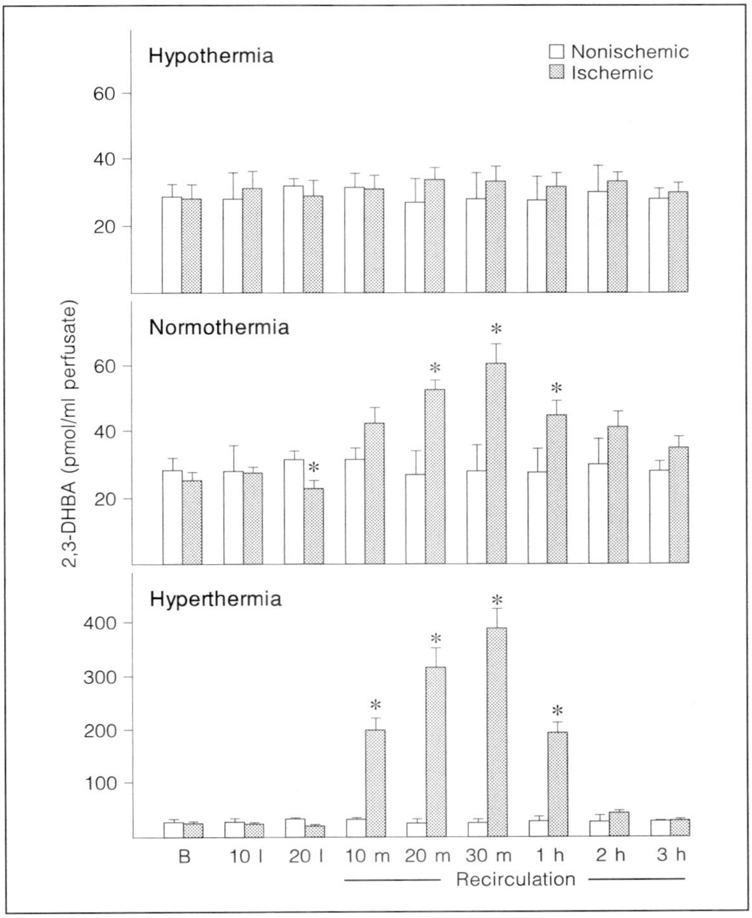

Fig. 3. Levels of 2,3-DHBA, denoting hydroxyl radical activity, in the striatal microdialysis perfusate of nonischemic rats and animals with 20 min of global forebrain ischemia under either hypothermic (30 °C), normothermic (37 °C), or hyperthermic (39 °C) conditions, followed in all cases by normothermic recirculation. The salicylate precursor was administered via the microdialysis probe. (Note that a 20-fold higher ordinate scale is used in the hyperthermia plot.) Data are means ± SEM. * Significantly different from nonischemic rats ($p < 0.05$). Reproduced from Globus et al. [63] with permission.

The 72-kD heat-shock protein HSP-72, along with related proteins, is induced by transient ischemia and may be neuroprotective [76]. However, the fact that HSP-72 is induced 48 h following 8 min of normothermic forebrain ischemia, but is not induced following hypothermic (30 °C) ischemia [77], suggests that heat-shock protein induction cannot be invoked to explain the neuroprotective effect of moderate hypothermia.

Another protein, uniquitin, binds to abnormal proteins produced by neural injury and facilitates their digestion by proteases [78]. In gerbils with 5 min ischemia, both normo- and hypothermic animals underwent loss of ubiquitin activity 6 h later, but the latter group showed subsequent restitution at 24–48 h; this enhanced postischemic resynthesis of ubiquitin may contribute to hypothermic neuroprotection [79].

Postischemic Hypothermia in Global Ischemia

A crucial investigative question, with broad clinical ramifications, is to what extent hypothermia is neuroprotective when applied *following* an hypoxic/ischemic insult. In a model of 10 min normothermic forebrain ischemia in rats by 'two-vessel' occlusion, we assessed the neuropathological sequelae of cranial hypothermia (30 °C) begun either at 5 or 30 min following the insult and maintained for 3 h [80]. Cooling begun at 5 min postinsult produced about 50% protection of hippocampal CA1 pyramidal neurons *when assessed at 3 days' survival*, whereas cooling begun at 30 min was ineffective. Other studies have shown that the duration of ischemia contributes to determining the therapeutic efficacy of postischemic cooling, i.e., cooling to 34 °C applied for 2 h following 8 min of normothermic ischemia partially protected, whereas when applied after 12 min of ischemia, it did not [31].

Dietrich et al. [81] subsequently raised the crucial issue of whether this degree of postischemic hypothermia was *permanently* protective and found that it was not: rats were given 10 min of normothermic ischemia followed immediately by 3 h cranial hypothermia to 30 °C, and were allowed to recover for either 3 days, 7 days, or 2 months prior to light microscopic histopathology. Hypothermic animals with 3-day survival showed (the expected) significant protection of CA1 pyramidal neurons, but this protective effect declined in the 7-day survivors and was lost in rats surviving 2 months [81] (fig. 4). (By contrast, rats cooled to 30 °C *during* ischemia were permanently protected at 2 months.) The key implications of this study are (a) that postischemic hypothermia markedly *delays*, but may not permanently prevent, ischemic neuronal injury, and (b) that chronic survival is therefore necessary when assessing permanent neuroprotection.

The above findings suggested that, by markedly delaying the process of neuronal death, postischemic hypothermia might broaden the therapeutic

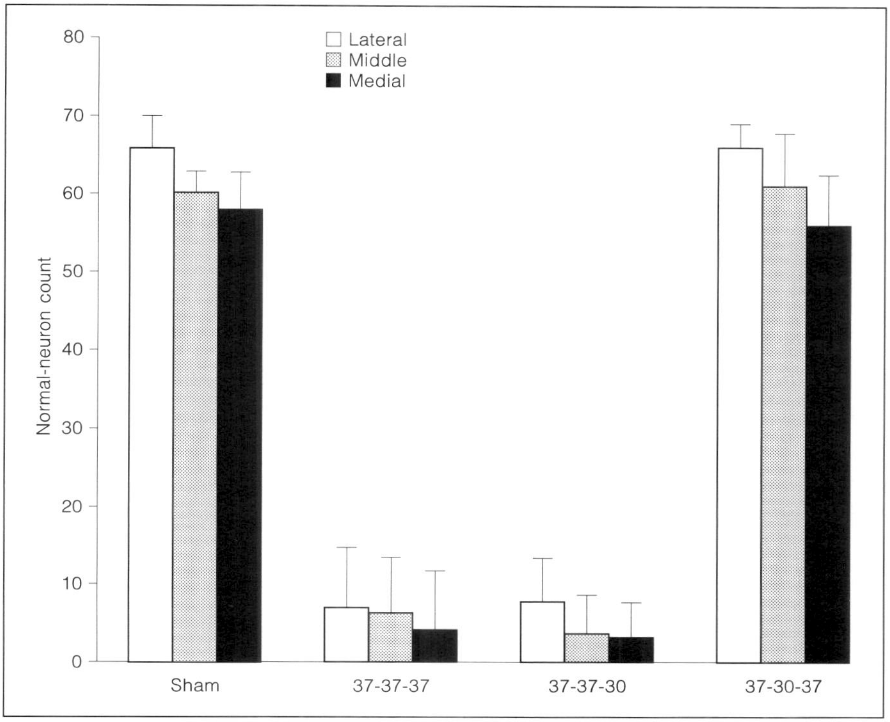

Fig. 4. Normal-neuron counts per high-power (× 400) microscopic field (means ± SD) in lateral, middle and medial hippocampal CA1 subsectors of rats with 10 min global forebrain ischemia followed by *2-month* survival. Sham-operated rats (Sham) have a normal complement of CA1 neurons. Rats which are normothermic throughout ischemia and recirculation (37-37-37), and rats with normothermic ischemia (37 °C) followed by postischemic cooling (30 °C for 3 h) (37-37-30) show greatly reduced neuronal counts ($p < 0.05$, ANOVA). By contrast, rats with *intraischemic* hypothermia (30 °C) (37-30-37) show essentially complete neuronal protection at 2 months. Replotted from the data of Dietrich et al. [81].

window for intervention with other, pharmacologic, neuroprotectants. This was tested in a paradigm involving 10 min global ischemia, 3 h immediate postischemic hypothermia to 30 °C, to which the NMDA antagonist MK-801 was first administered on days 3, 5, and 7 postischemia; the addition of MK-801 to postischemic hypothermia conferred permanent partial protection on CA1 neurons which would have succumbed with hypothermia alone [82]. This combined-treatment paradigm also provided protection from ischemia-associated behavioral placing task deficits [83]. These findings may have important clinical ramifications in the design of clinical neuroprotectant trials.

Others have shown that *longer* periods of postischemic cooling tend to confer more permanent neuroprotection. Thus, 24-hour cooling to 32 °C commencing 1 h following 5 min global ischemia in gerbils resulted in about 90% preservation of CA1 neurons, which would otherwise have been largely lost [84]. Even with 6-month survival, about 70% of CA1 neurons remain rescued [85]. These studies show that postischemic cooling is capable of providing long-lasting neuroprotection but that this depends upon the delay in initiating therapy, its duration, and the extent of cooling [85].

Hypothermic Mediation of Putative 'Pharmacologic' Neuroprotection
Important studies have shown that, unless temperature is carefully monitored and controlled, neuroprotective effects may be falsely ascribed to pharmacologic agents which act by producing inadvertent hypothermia. This was the case with the NMDA antagonist MK-801 (dizocilpine), which was initially reported to be highly protective in global ischemia in some [e.g., 86] but not other studies [87]. A careful reassessment of this problem revealed that the observed neuroprotective effect of MK-801 occurred in conjunction with a prolonged period of hypothermia [88]; when normothermia was maintained, the protective effect was lost [88, 89]. (Interestingly, the obverse of this has been shown in focal ischemia, in which MK-801 is ordinarily neuroprotective; by allowing temperature to rise to 39.0–39.5 °C during ischemia, however, the protective effect of MK-801 is lost [90].)

Hypothermic Neuroprotection in Focal Cerebral Ischemia – Permanent vs. Temporary MCA Occlusion

We assessed hypothermic neuroprotection in Sprague-Dawley rats with proximal MCA clip occlusion by reducing brain temperature to 30 °C for 2 h, and evaluating infarct volume histologically at 3 days [91]. Significant neuroprotection was seen in rats with 2-hour periods of *temporary* MCA occlusion, in which intraischemic cooling reduced cortical infarct volume by about 70%, and striatal infarct volume by about 50%. By contrast, the same cooling paradigm, when applied to rats with *permanent* MCA occlusion, appeared to modify the topographic distribution of infarction somewhat, without significantly reducing infarct volume. Importantly, the opposite was observed with mild *hyperthermia* (39 vs. 36 °C during the 2-hour MCA occlusion period) i.e., a 3-fold *increase* in infarct volume.

An important mechanism contributing to deterioration of the ischemic penumbra and the growth of a focal infarct is the occurrence of repetitive cortical depolarizations [e.g., see 92]. Intraischemic hypothermia (30 °C) suppresses these depolarizations and, pari passu, reduces infarct volume, while intraischemic hyperthermia (40 °C; see below) increases numbers of DC potential deflections and increases infarct size [93].

In a recent review [94], we considered the factors which determine the extent of hypothermic neuroprotection in focal ischemia (table 1). The most pronounced therapeutic effect, amounting to an infarct size reduction of over 90%, was observed in *temporary* (3 h) MCA occlusion in which cooling (to 32 °C) was begun at the onset of ischemia and maintained for several hours [96]. Even when hypothermia is delayed by 3 h, significant protection has been observed when cooling to 30–32 °C has been maintained for several hours [96, 101]. Models of *permanent* vascular occlusion are in general more resistant to hypothermic neuroprotection, but infarct size reductions of about 80% have been reported in such models with profound cooling (24–32 °C) instituted immediately after ischemia [98, 100] (table 1). Other studies confirm treatment success with delays of 1–2 h [96, 98, 103], particularly if the cooling period is prolonged [103]. Other studies, however, suggest that the window of efficacy is narrower [105]. It would thus appear from these studies, taken together, that the therapeutic effect of hypothermia in focal ischemia is more pronounced in temporary than in permanent vascular occlusion; that the intensity and duration of cooling affect the extent of therapeutic response, and that the therapeutic effect is *graded*, with progressive loss of therapeutic benefit as treatment is delayed or made less intense. The therapeutic window for hypothermia in focal ischemia may begin to close by 1–3 h poststroke [94] (table 1).

Therapeutic Hypothermia in Related Conditions

Moderate hypothermia (30–33 °C) instituted during or shortly after fluid-percussion traumatic brain injury (TBI) in rats has also been found to be significantly neuroprotective, when assessed both behaviorally and neuropathologically [106–108], and hypothermia has been shown to attenuate the increase of interleukin-1β, a proinflammatory cytokine which otherwise rises following TBI [109]. These observations have led to the use of hypothermia in patients with severe closed head injury [110] and have spawned a clinical randomized trial of systemic hypothermia (32–33 °C for 48 h) in this condition [111]. Results were encouraging, and a phase III multicenter trial is currently in progress. Techniques have been developed for measuring intracerebral temperature directly in neurosurgical patients [110, 112, 113], and brain > rectal temperature gradients have been observed. Episodic cerebral hyperthermia has been noted in head-injured patients during extended monitoring, providing a

Table 1. Therapeutic hypothermia in focal cerebral ischemia in the rat: influence of model, and of duration, intensity, and delay in initiation of cooling [modified from 24]

Reference	Model	Rat strain	Duration of ischemia	Temperature °C	Initiation of cooling	Duration of cooling	Survival time	Infarct size % control
Morikawa et al. [91]	MCA-ct + HT	SD	Perm	30 (36) b	0 h	4 h	3 d	98% ctx
	MCA-ct	SD	Perm	30 (36) b	0 h	2 h	3 d	74% ctx,*
	MCA-clp	SD	2 h	30 (36) b	0 h	2 h	3 d	28% ctx
Ridenour et al. [95]	MCA-lig	SHR	Perm	33 (37) c	0 h	2 h	4 d	94% hem
	MCA-lig	SHR	1 h	33 (37) c	0 h	2 h	4 d	52% hem,*
Xue et al. [96]	MCA/bpCCA	Wis	Perm	32 (37) r	0 h	6 h	6 h	39% ctx,*
	MCA/btCCA	Wis	3 h	32 (37) r	0 h	3 h	1 d	8% ctx,*
	MCA/btCCA	Wis	3 h	32 (37) r	0 h	1.5 h	1 d	55% ctx,*
	MCA/btCCA	Wis	3 h	32 (37) r	1.5 h	1.5 h	1 d	51% ctx,*
	MCA/btCCA	Wis	3 h	32 (37) r	1.5 h	3 h	1 d	27% ctx,*
	MCA/btCCA	Wis	3 h	32 (37) r	0 h	3 h	3 d	16% ctx,*
	MCA/btCCA	Wis	3 h	32 (37) r	3 h	3 h	6 h	39% ctx,*
Chen et al. [97]	MCA-sut	Wis	2 h	30 (37) r	0 h	3 h	4 d	small size, hem
Baker et al. [98]	MCA-ct	Wis	Perm	24 (36) r	0 h	1 h	1 d	20% hem,*
	MCA-ct	Wis	Perm	24 (36) r	0.5 h	1 h	1 d	41% hem,*
	MCA-ct	Wis	Perm	24 (36) r	1 h	1 h	1 d	33% hem,*
	MCA-ct	Wis	Perm	24 (36) r	2 h	1 h	1 d	158% hem,(*)
	MCA-ct	Wis	Perm	24 (36) r	3 h	1 h	1 d	110% hem
Kader et al. [99]	MCA/ipCCA	Wis	Perm	30 (37) c	0 h	1 h	1 d	47% hem,*
	MCA/ipCCA	Wis	Perm	33 (37) c	0 h	1 h	1 d	42% hem,*
	MCA/ipCCA	Wis	Perm	34.5 (37) c	0 h	1 h	1 d	43% hem,*
	MCA/ipCCA	Wis	Perm	33 (37) c	1 h	1 h	1 d	46% hem,*
Moyer et al. [100]	MCA/bttCCA	Wis	Perm	32-sp (37) b	0 h	1 h	1 d	23% ctx,*
	MCA/bttCCA	Wis	Perm	32 (37) b	40 min	1 h	1 d	91% ctx
Zhang et al. [101]	MCA-sut	Wis	2 h	30 (37) r	3 h	3 h	7 d	53% hem,*
Goto et al. [102]	MCA/btCCA	SD	3 h	33 (36) c	0 h	3 h	3 d	78% hem,*
	MCA/btCCA	SD	3 h	28 (36) c	0 h	3 h	3 d	50% hem,*
Zhang et al. [103]	MCA-sut	Wis	2 h	30 (37) r	2 h	1 h	7 d	89% hem
	MCA-sut	Wis	2 h	30 (37) r	2 h	3 h	7 d	16% hem,*

Table 1 (continued)

Reference	Model	Rat strain	Duration of ischemia	Temperature °C	Initiation of cooling	Duration of cooling	Survival time	Infarct size % control
Karibe et al. [104]	MCA-sut	SD	2 h	32-3 (37) b	10 min pre	2 h	1 d	2% ctx,*
	MCA-sut	SD	2 h	32-3 (37) b	10 min	1.8 h	1 d	11% ctx,*
	MCA-sut	SD	2 h	32-3 (37) b	0.5 h	1.5 h	1 d	30% ctx,*
	MCA-sut	SD	2 h	32-3 (37) b	1 h	1 h	1 d	69% ctx (ns)
Markarian et al. [105]	MCA/bttCCA	SD	3 h	32-3 (36-7) c	0 h	1 h	3 d	102% hem
	MCA/bttCCA	SD	3 h	32-3 (36-7) c	0 h	2 h	3 d	92% hem
	MCA/bttCCA	SD	3 h	32-3 (36-7) c	0 h	3 h	3 d	81% hem,*
	MCA/bttCCA	SD	3 h	32-3 (36-7) c	0 h	4 h	3 d	80% hem,*
	MCA/bttCCA	SD	3 h	32-3 (36-7) c	0 h	3 h	3 d	81% hem,*
	MCA/bttCCA	SD	3 h	32-3 (36-7) c	0.25 h	3 h	3 d	82% hem,*
	MCA/bttCCA	SD	3 h	32-3 (36-7) c	0.5 h	3 h	3 d	85% hem,*
	MCA/bttCCA	SD	3 h	32-3 (36-7) c	0.75 h	3 h	3 d	98% hem

Model

MCA = middle cerebral artery occlusion; ct = produced by electrocautery; clp = produced by clip; lig = produced by ligation; sut = produced by intraluminal suture filament; HT = hypotension.

CCA = common carotid artery occlusion; ip = permanent ipsilateral occlusion; bt = bilateral occlusions (ipsilateral permanent, contralateral temporary); btt = bilateral temporary occlusions; bp = bilateral permanent occlusions.

Rat strain

SD = Sprague-Dawley; Wis = Wistar; SHR = spontaneously hypertensive rat.

Duration of ischemia

Refers to duration of MCA occlusion (hours); Perm = permanent.

Temperature

Denotes temperature (°C) during therapeutic cooling period: b = measured in the brain; c = measured pericranially (e.g., temporalis muscle); r = measured rectally; sp = temperature allowed to fall spontaneously during ischemia; () = temperature of controls.

Initiation of cooling

Time at which cooling begun with reference to onset of MCA occlusion.

Infarct size

Expressed as percentage of control value: ctx = neocortex; hem = cerebral hemisphere; * = significantly different from normothermic control.

rationale for the rigorous avoidance of temperature elevations in the injured brain (see discussion of hyperthermia, below).

Mild-to-moderate hypothermia has also been used with success in experimental models of spinal cord ischemia [114], neonatal hypoxia-ischemia [115], and even in in vitro studies of oxygen-glucose deprivation in cortical cell culture [116].

Hyperthermia

An important by-product of recent studies on mild-to-moderate hypothermia has been the conclusive recognition that mild brain *hyperthermia* is strikingly deleterious when superimposed on the ischemic or injured brain. Thus, in our initial studies, mild brain warming to 39 °C during 20 min global ischemia led to severe ischemic changes in cortex, striatum and hippocampus, with focal thalamic injury [25]. A careful study comparing intraischemic brain temperatures of 37 and 39 °C during 20 min global ischemia showed both an *acceleration* and a marked *accentuation and spread* of injury in the 39 °C group, in which severe neuronal injury was evident even at 1-day survival, with severe ischemic changes in striatum and hippocampal CA1 sector, laminar necrosis of cortex, foci of infarction in thalamus, and ischemic changes in cerebellum, pars reticulata of substantia nigra, and dentate granule cells of hippocampus [117]. These observations have been amply confirmed in the rat [30] and gerbil [71]. Merely blunting the mild (1.5 °C) hyperthermia which occurs during the first 90 min following a 5-min period of global ischemia in gerbils is sufficient to reduce markedly the degree of CA1 pyramidal neuron loss which would otherwise occur [118].

Recent studies have investigated possible mechanisms of hyperthermic exacerbation of injury. Striatal microdialysis sampling in rats with 20 min forebrain ischemia have shown higher levels of glutamate release in rats with raised intraischemic brain temperature (39 °C, as opposed to 37 °C), along with a trend toward higher persistent glutamate levels during the recirculation period, and persistently elevated glycine levels [119]. The excitotoxic index, a composite descriptor of excitatory/inhibitory neurotransmitter imbalance, was only 2-fold elevated in the 37 °C group, but increased by 20-fold during recirculation in rats with 39 °C ischemia [119]. A similar phenomenon occurs in focal ischemia (MCA occlusion in rats), in which release of glutamate in the cortical ischemic penumbra attains almost 7-fold higher peaks during 2 h hyperthermic MCA occlusion (39 °C) than during the corresponding normothermic insult [120].

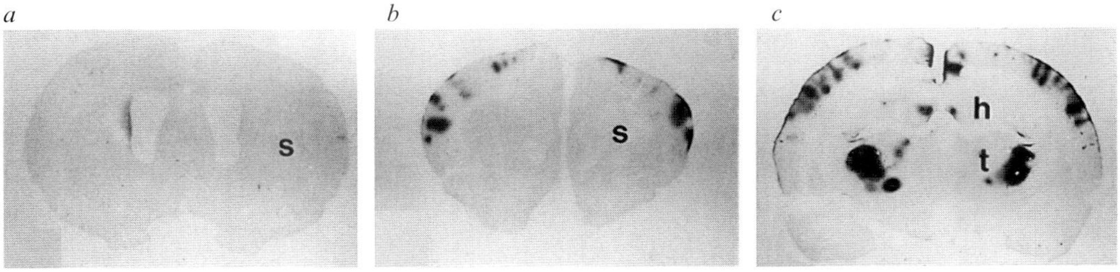

Fig. 5. Cleared vibratome sections reacted for horseradish peroxidase (HRP-O/L) histochemistry at 45–60 min following a 20-min period of global forebrain ischemia at intraischemic brain temperatures of 33 (*a*), 36 (*b*), or 39 °C (*c*). The brain which was ischemic at 33 °C (*a*) shows HRP leakage only adjacent to lateral ventricle. Ischemia at 36 °C (*b*) leads to protein extravasation at cortical sites but not striatum (s). With ischemia at 39 °C (*c*), there is widespread extravasation of HRP in cortex and thalamus (t) as well as hippocampus (h). Reproduced from Dietrich et al. [121] with permission.

Microdialysis studies have shown that intraischemic hyperthermia (39 °C) during global ischemia markedly potentiates the production of hydroxyl radicals (by 4- to 5-fold) compared to normothermic ischemia (fig. 3) [63, 64] – the opposite of the phenomenon observed with hypothermic ischemia (see discussion above).

The blood-brain barrier (BBB) is particularly vulnerable to hyperthermic ischemia (and is protected by hypothermia) (fig. 5). Following 20 min of forebrain ischemia at 30 or 33 °C, the barrier is intact to horseradish peroxidase administered during the early recirculation period. In contrast, rats with ischemia at 37 °C show small cortical foci of BBB breakdown and rats with 39 °C ischemia show strikingly widespread protein extravasation throughout cortical as well as subcortical structures [121]. These foci of BBB disruption correlate with, and thus might contribute to, sites of neuronal cell death [122].

Recent studies from our laboratory in rat models of both global [123] and focal ischemia [124] show that hyperthermia need not be immediate: even when transiently instituted 24 h following an ischemic insult, elevated brain temperatures (39–40 °C) are capable of markedly exacerbating the resulting injury. These observations, taken together, should constitute a stern warning to clinicians *to suppress even mild fever* in patients with acute ischemic or traumatic injury, to avoid secondary injury, and to avoid cerebral hyperthermia during rewarming following cardiopulmonary bypass procedures [125].

Concluding Recommendations

Experimental studies of mild-to-moderate brain temperature manipulations in the settings of ischemia and injury have yielded a sufficient body of information that we can, with some assurance, offer the following recommendations. (See also Maher and Hachinski [126] for a recent summary of these matters.)

(a) Given an overwhelming body of experimental evidence that even mild degrees of *hyper*thermia severely exacerbate the outcome of brain ischemia or trauma, clinicians should vigorously combat even minor fevers in patients with stroke or CNS injury. In fact, a very recent prospective study of 390 patients admitted to hospital within 6 h of ischemic stroke has shown lower mortality and improved outcome (measured at discharge on the Scandinavian Stroke Scale) in patients with mild hypothermia on admission, and higher mortality and worse outcome in hyperthermic patients [127]. Body temperature was independently related to infarct size and outcome with a high degree of statistical significance.

(b) Without question, the time has come for a multicenter, prospective, randomized trial of moderate systemic cooling (e.g., 33–34 °C) in acute ischemic stroke. Clinician-scientists should be urged to initiate this type of investigation. As noted above, such a phase III study, supported by the National Institutes of Health, is now in progress for acute head trauma.

(c) As moderate hypothermia following global ischemia *delays* the onset of ischemic histopathological alterations, we predict that hypothermia may extend the therapeutic window for pharmacologic neuroprotection and, as such, play an important role in conjunction with neuroprotective drugs in the treatment of acute cerebral ischemia [82]. A possible adjunctive role of hypothermia in acute thrombolytic therapy also deserves further study. Interestingly, recent work on this subject has confirmed that *hyper*thermia is detrimental when combined with thrombolysis and thus should be avoided [128].

References

1 Smith LW, Fay T: Temperature factors in cancer and embryonal cell growth. JAMA 1939;113:653–660.

2 Fay T: Observations on generalized refrigeration in cases of severe cerebral trauma. Assoc Res Nerv Ment Dis Proc 1943;24:611–619.

3 Fay T, Smith GW: Observations on reflex responses during prolonged periods of human refrigeration. Arch Neurol Psychiatry 1941;45:215–222.

4 Berger RL: Nazi science – The Dachau hypothermia experiments. N Engl J Med 1990;322:1435–1446.

5 Sealy WC, Brown IW Jr, Young WG Jr: A report on the use of both extracorporeal circulation and hypothermia for open heart surgery. Ann Surg 1958;147:603–613.

6 Botterell EH, Lougheed WM, Scott JW, Vandewater SL: Hypothermia, and interruption of carotid, or carotid and vertebral circulation, in the surgical management of intracranial aneurysms. J Neurosurg 1956;13:1–42.
7 Spetzler RF, Hadley MN, Rigamonti D, Carter LP, Raudzens PA, Shedd SA, Wilkinson E: Aneurysms of the basilar artery treated with circulatory arrest, hypothermia, and barbiturate cerebral protection. J Neurosurg 1988;68:868–879.
8 Pontius RG, Brockman HL, Hardy EG, Cooley DA, DeBakey ME: The use of hypothermia in the prevention of paraplegia following temporary aortic occlusion: Experimental observations. Surgery 1954;36:33–38.
9 Ginsberg MD, Sternau LL, Globus MY-T, Dietrich WD, Busto R: Therapeutic modulation of brain temperature: Relevance to ischemic brain injury. Cerebrovasc Brain Metab Rev 1992;4:189–225.
10 Rosomoff HL, Holaday DA: Cerebral blood flow and cerebral oxygen consumption during hypothermia. Am J Physiol 1954;179:85–88.
11 Rosomoff HL, Gilbert R: Brain volume and cerebrospinal fluid pressure during hypothermia. Am J Physiol 1955;183:19–22.
12 Michenfelder JD, Van Dyke RA, Theye RA: The effects of anesthetic agents and techniques on canine cerebral ATP and lactate levels. Anesthesiology 1970;33:315–321.
13 Hagerdal M, Harp J, Nilsson L, Siesjö BK: The effect of induced hypothermia upon oxygen comsumption in the rat brain. J Neurochem 1975;24:311–316.
14 Rosomoff HL: Hypothermia and cerebral vascular lesions. I. Experimental interruption of the middle cerebral artery during hypothermia. J Neurosurg 1956;13:332–343.
15 Rosomoff HL: Hypothermia and cerebral vascular lesions. II. Experimental middle cerebral artery interruption followed by induction of hypothermia. AMA Arch Neurol Psychiatry 1957;78:454–464.
16 Rosomoff HL: Experimental brain injury during hypothermia. J Neurosurg 1959;16:177–187.
17 Connolly JE, Boyd RJ, Calvin JW: The protective effect of hypothermia in cerebral ischemia: Experimental and clinical application by selective brain cooling in the human. Surgery 1962;52: 15–24.
18 Ommaya AK, Baldwin M: Direct extravascular brain cooling in the normothermic animal. Neurology 1962;12:882–895.
19 White RJ, Massopust LA Jr, Wolin LR, Taslitz N, Yashon D: Profound selective cooling and ischemia of primate brain without pump or oxygenator. Surgery 1969;66:224–232.
20 Hirsch H, Müller HA: Funktionelle und histologische Veränderungen des Kaninchengehirns nach kompletter Gehirnischämie. Pflügers Arch 1962;275:277–291.
21 Hagerdal M, Welsh FA, Keykhah M, Perez E, Harp JR: Protective effects of combinations of hypothermia and barbiturates in cerebral hypoxia in the rat. Anesthesiology 1978;49:165–169.
22 Berntman L, Welsh FA, Harp JR: Cerebral protective effect of low-grade hypothermia. Anesthesiology 1981;55:495–498.
23 Smith M-L, Auer RN, Siesjö BK: The density and distribution of ischemic brain injury in the rat following 2–10 min of forebrain ischemia. Acta Neuropathol (Berl) 1984;64:319–332.
24 Vibulsresth S, Dietrich WD, Busto R, Ginsberg MD: Failure of nimodipine to prevent ischemic neuronal damage in rats. Stroke 1987;18:210–216.
25 Busto R, Dietrich WD, Globus MY-T, Valdes I, Scheinberg P, Ginsberg MD: Small differences in intraischemic brain temperature critically determine the extent of ischemic neuronal injury. J Cereb Blood Flow Metab 1987;7:729–738.
26 Busto R, Dietrich WD, Globus MY-T, Ginsberg MD: The importance of brain temperature in cerebral ischemic injury. Stroke 1989;20:1113–1114.
27 Pulsinelli WA, Brierley JB: A new model of bilateral hemispheric ischemia in the unanesthetized rat. Stroke 1979;10:267–272.
28 Minamisawa H, Nordström C-H, Smith M-L, Siesjö BK: The influence of mild body and brain hypothermia on ischemic brain damage. J Cereb Blood Flow Metab 1990;10:365–374.
29 Minamisawa H, Mellergard P, Smith M-L, Bengtsson F, Theander S, Boris-Möller F, Siesjö BK: Preservation of brain temperature during ischemia in rats. Stroke 1990;21:758–764.
30 Minamisawa H, Smith M-L, Siesjö BK: The effect of mild hyperthermia and hypothermia on brain damage following 5, 10, and 15 minutes of forebrain ischemia. Ann Neurol 1990;28:26–33.

31 Chopp M, Chen H, Dereski MO, Garcia JH: Mild hypothermic intervention after graded ischemic stress in rats. Stroke 1991;22:37–43.

32 Freund TF, Buzsaki G, Leon A, Somogyi P: Hippocampal cell death following ischemia: Effects of brain temperature and anesthesia. Exp Neurol 1990;108:251–260.

33 Lundgren J, Smith M-L, Siesjö BK: Influence of moderate hypothermia on ischemic brain damage incurred under hyperglycemic conditions. Exp Brain Res 1991;84:91–101.

34 Leonov Y, Sterz F, Safar P, Radovsky A, Oku K-i, Tisherman S, Stezoski SW: Mild cerebral hypothermia during and after cardiac arrest improves neurologic outcome in dogs. J Cereb Blood Flow Metab 1990;10:57–70.

35 Weinrauch V, Safar P, Tisherman S, Kuboyama K, Radovsky A: Beneficial effect of mild hypothermia and detrimental effect of deep hypothermia after cardiac arrest in dogs. Stroke 1992;23:1454–1462.

36 Kuboyama K, Safar P, Radovsky A, Tisherman SA, Stezoski SW, Alexander H: Delay in cooling negates the beneficial effect of mild resuscitative cerebral hypothermia after cardiac arrest in dogs: A prospective, randomized study. Crit Care Med 1993;21:1348–1358.

37 Wass CT, Lanier WL, Hofer RE, Scheithauer BW, Andrews AG: Temperature changes of $\geqslant 1$ °C alter functional neurologic outcome and histopathology in a canine model of complete cerebral ischemia. Anesthesiology 1995;83:325–335.

38 Busto R, Globus MY-T, Dietrich WD, Martinez E, Valdés I, Ginsberg MD: Effect of mild hypothermia on ischemia-induced release of neurotransmitters and free fatty acids in rat brain. Stroke 1989;20:904–910.

39 Welsh FA, Sims RE, Harris VA: Mild hypothermia prevents ischemic injury in gerbil hippocampus. J Cereb Blood Flow Metab 1990;10:557–563.

40 Michenfelder JD, Theye RA: The effects of anesthesia and hypothermia on canine cerebral ATP and lactate during anoxia produced by decapitation. Anesthesiology 1970;33:430–439.

41 Natale JE, D'Alecy LG: Protection from cerebral ischemia by brain cooling without reduced lactate accumulation in dogs. Stroke 1989;20:770–777.

42 Chopp M, Knight R, Tidwell CD, Helpern JA, Brown E, Welch KMA: The metabolic effects of mild hypothermia on global cerebral ischemia and recirculation in the cat: Comparison to normothermia and hyperthermia. J Cereb Blood Flow Metab 1989;9:141–148.

43 Ginsberg MD, Busto R, Martinez E, Globus MY-T, Valdés I, Loor JY: The effects of cerebral ischemia on energy metabolism; in Schousboe A, Diemer NH, Kofod H (eds): Drug Research Related to Neuroactive Amino Acids – Alfred Benzon Symposium 32. Copenhagen, Munksgaard, 1992, pp 207–224.

44 Ginsberg MD, Busto R, Castella Y, Valdes I, Loor J: The protective effect of moderate intraischemic brain hypothermia is associated with improved postischemic glucose utilization and blood flow. J Cereb Blood Flow Metab 1989;9(suppl 1):S380.

45 Dietrich WD, Busto R, Alonso O, Pita-Loor Y, Globus MY-T, Ginsberg MD: Intraischemic brain hypothermia promotes postischemic metabolic recovery and somatosensory circuit activation. J Cereb Blood Flow Metab 1991;11(suppl 2):S846.

46 Green EJ, Dietrich WD, van Dijk F, Busto R, Markgraf CG, McCabe PM, Ginsberg MD, Schneiderman N: Protective effects of brain hypothermia on histopathology and behavior following global cerebral ischemia in rats. Brain Res 1992;580:197–204.

47 Widmann R, Miyazawa T, Hossmann K-A: Protective effect of hypothermia on hippocampal injury after 30 minutes of forebrain ischemia in rats is mediated by postischemic recovery of protein synthesis. J Neurochem 1993;61:200–209.

48 Benveniste H: The excitotoxin hypothesis in relation to cerebral ischemia. Cerebrovasc Brain Metab Rev 1991;3:213–245.

49 Globus MY-T, Busto R, Dietrich WD, Martinez E, Valdés I, Ginsberg MD: Effect of ischemia on the in vivo release of striatal dopamine, glutamate, and gamma-aminobutyric acid studied by intracerebral microdialysis. J Neurochem 1988;51:1455–1464.

50 Okuda C, Saito A, Miyazaki M, Kuriyama K: Alteration of the turnover of dopamine and 5-hydroxytryptamine in rat brain associated with hypothermia. Pharmacol Biochem Behav 1986;25:79–83.

51 Graf R, Matsumoto K, Risse F, Rosner G, Heiss W-D: Effect of mild hypothermia on glutamate accumulation in cat focal ischemia. Stroke 1992;23:150.
52 Globus MY-T, Busto R, Dietrich WD, Martinez E, Valdés I, Ginsberg MD: Intraischemic extracellular release of dopamine and glutamate is associated with striatal vulnerability to ischemia. Neurosci Lett 1988;91:36–40.
53 Mitani A, Kataoka K: Critical levels of extracellular glutamate mediating gerbil hippocampal delayed neuronal death during hypothermia: Brain microdialysis study. Neuroscience 1991;42:661–670.
54 Baker AJ, Zornow MH, Grafe MR, Scheller MS, Skilling SR, Smullin DH, Larson AA: Hypothermia prevents ischemia-induced increases in hippocampal glycine concentrations in rabbits. Stroke 1991; 22:666–673.
55 Choi DW, Maulucci-Gedde M, Kriegstein AR: Glutamate neurotoxicity in cortical cell culture. J Neurosci 1987;7:357–368.
56 Rothman SM, Olney JW: Glutamate and the pathophysiology of hypoxic-ischemic brain damage. Ann Neurol 1986;19:105–111.
57 Choi DW, Rothman SM: The role of glutamate neurotoxicity in hypoxic-ischemic neuronal death. Annu Rev Neurosci 1990;13:171–182.
58 Albers GW, Goldberg MP, Choi DW: N-methyl-*D*-aspartate antagonists: Ready for clinical trial in brain ischemia? Ann Neurol 1989;25:398–403.
59 Globus MY-T, Ginsberg MD, Harik SI, Busto R, Dietrich WD: Role of dopamine in ischemic striatal injury: Metabolic evidence. Neurology 1987;37:1712–1719.
60 Globus MY-T, Ginsberg MD, Busto R: Excitotoxic index – A biochemical marker of selective vulnerability. Neurosci Lett 1991;127:39–42.
61 Globus MY-T, Busto R, Martinez E, Valdés I, Dietrich WD, Ginsberg MD: Comparative effect of transient global ischemia on extracellular levels of glutamate, glycine, and gamma-aminobutyric acid in vulnerable and nonvulnerable brain regions in the rat. J Neurochem 1991;57:470–478.
62 Globus MY-T, Busto R, Martinez E, Valdés I, Dietrich MD, Ginsberg MD: Early moderate postischemic hypothermia attenuates the rise in excitotoxic index in the hippocampus – A possible mechanism for the beneficial effects of early postischemic moderate cooling. J Cereb Blood Flow Metab 1991;11(suppl 2):S10
63 Globus MY-T, Busto R, Lin B, Schnippering H, Ginsberg MD: Detection of free radical activity during transient global ischemia and recirculation: Effects of intraischemic brain temperature modulation. J Neurochem 1995;65:1250–1256.
64 Kil HY, Zhang J, Piantadosi CA: Brain temperature alters hydroxyl radical production during cerebral ischemia/reperfusion in rats. J Cereb Blood Flow Metab 1996;16:100–106.
65 Morimoto T, Globus MY-T, Busto R, Martinez E, Ginsberg MD: Simultaneous measurement of salicylate hydroxylation and glutamate release in the penumbral cortex following transient middle cerebral artery occlusion in rats. J Cereb Blood Flow Metab 1996;16:92–99.
66 Globus MY-T, Alonso O, Dietrich WD, Busto R, Ginsberg MD: Glutamate release and free radical production following brain injury: Effects of posttraumatic hypothermia. J Neurochem 1995;65: 1704–1711.
67 Karibe H, Chen SF, Zarow GJ, Gafni J, Graham SH, Chan PH, Weinstein PR: Mild intraischemic hypothermia suppresses consumption of endogenous antioxidants after temporary focal ischemia in rats. Brain Res 1994;649:12–18.
68 Kader A, Frazzini VI, Baker CJ, Solomon RA, Trifiletti RR: Effect of mild hypothermia on nitric oxide synthesis during focal cerebral ischemia. Neurosurgery 1994;35:272–277.
69 Llinas R, McGuinness TL, Leonard CS, Sugimori M, Greengard P: Intraterminal injection of synapsin I or calcium-calmodulin-dependent protein kinase II alters neurotransmitter release at the squid giant synapse. Proc Natl Acad Sci USA 1985;82:3035–3039.
70 Taft WC, Tennes-Rees KA, Blair RE, Clifton GL, DeLorenzo RJ: Cerebral ischemia decreases endogenous calcium-dependent protein phosphorylation in gerbil brain. Brain Res 1988;447:159–163.
71 Churn SB, Taft WC, Billingsley MS, Blair RE, DeLorenzo RJ: Temperature modulation of ischemic neuronal death and inhibition of calcium/calmodulin-dependent protein kinase II in gerbils. Stroke 1990;21:1715–1721.

72 Nishizuka Y: Studies and perspectives of protein kinase C. Science 1986;233:305–312.
73 Wieloch T, Cardell M, Bingren H, Zivin J, Saitoh T: Changes in the activity of protein kinase C and the differential subcellular redistribution of its isozymes in the rat striatum during and folowing transient forebrain ischemia. J Neurochem 1991;56:1227–1235.
74 Cardell M, Boris-Möller F, Wieloch T: Hypothermia prevents the ischemia-induced translocation and inhibition of protein kinase C in the rat striatum. J Neurochem 1991;57:1814–1817.
75 Busto R, Globus MY-T, Neary JT, Ginsberg MD: Regional alterations of protein kinase C activity following transient cerebral ischemia: Effects of intraischemic brain temperature modulation. J Neurochem 1994;63:1095–1103.
76 Barbe MF, Tytell M, Gower DJ, Welch WJ: Hyperthermia protects against light damage in the rat retina. Science 1988;241:1817–1820.
77 Chopp M, Li Y, Dereski MO, Levine SR, Yoshida Y, Garcia JH: Hypothermia reduces 72 kD heat-shock protein induction in rat brain after transient forebrain ischemia. Stroke 1992;23:104–107.
78 Rechsteiner M: Ubiquitin mediated pathways for intracellular proteolysis. Annu Rev Cell Biol 1987; 3:1–30.
79 Yamashita K, Eguchi Y, Kajiwara K, Ito H: Mild hypothermia ameliorates ubiquitin synthesis and prevents delayed neuronal death in the gerbil hippocampus. Stroke 1991;22:1574–1581.
80 Busto R, Dietrich WD, Globus MY-T, Ginsberg MD: Postischemic moderate hypothermia inhibits CA1 hippocampal ischemic neuronal injury. Neurosci Lett 1989;101:299–304.
81 Dietrich WD, Busto R, Alonso O, Globus MY-T, Ginsberg MD: Intraischemic but not postischemic brain hypothermia protects chronically following global forebrain ischemia in rats. J Cereb Blood Flow Metab 1993;13:541–549.
82 Dietrich WD, Lin B, Globus MY-T, Green EJ, Ginsberg MD, Busto R: Effect of delayed MK-801 (dizocilpine) treatment with or without immediate postischemic hypothermia on chronic neuronal survival after global forebrain ischemia in rats. J Cereb Blood Flow Metab 1995;15:960–968.
83 Green EJ, Pazos AJ, Dietrich WD, McCabe PM, Schneiderman N, Lin B, Busto R, et al: Combined postischemic hypothermia and delayed MK-801 treatment attenuates neurobehavioral deficits associated with transient global ischemia in rats. Brain Res 1995;702:145–152.
84 Colbourne F, Corbett D: Delayed and prolonged post-ischemic hypothermia is neuroprotective in the gerbil. Brain Res 1994;654:265–272.
85 Colbourne F, Corbett D: Delayed postischemic hypothermia: A six-month survival study using behavioral and histological assessments of neuroprotection. J Neurosci 1995;15:7250–7260.
86 Gill R, Foster AC, Woodruff GN: MK-801 is neuroprotective in gerbils when administered during the post-ischaemic period. Neuroscience 1988;25:847–855.
87 Buchan AM: Do NMDA antagonists protect against cerebral ischemia? Are clinical trials warranted? Cerebrovasc Brain Metab Rev 1990;2:1–26.
88 Buchan A, Pulsinelli WA: Hypothermia but not the N-methyl-*D*-aspartate antagonist MK-801 attenuates neuronal damage in gerbils subjected to transient global ischemia. J Neurosci 1990;10:311–316.
89 Buchan A, Li H, Pulsinelli WA: The N-methyl-*D*-aspartate antagonist, MK-801, fails to protect against neuronal damage caused by transient, severe forebrain ischemia in adult rats. J Neurosci 1991;11:1049–1056.
90 Memezawa H, Zhao Q, Smith M-L, Siesjö BK: Hyperthermia nullifies the ameliorating effect of dizocilpine maleate (MK-801) in focal cerebral ischemia. Brain Res 1995;670:48–52.
91 Morikawa E, Ginsberg MD, Dietrich WD, Duncan RC, Kraydieh S, Globus MY-T, Busto R: The significance of brain temperature in focal cerebral ischemia: Histopathological consequences of middle cerebral artery occlusion in the rat. J Cereb Blood Flow Metab 1992;12:380–389.
92 Back T, Ginsberg MD, Dietrich WD, Watson BD: Induction of spreading depression in the ischemic hemisphere following experimental middle cerebral artery occlusion: Effect on infarct morphology. J Cereb Blood Flow Metab 1996;16:202–213.
93 Chen Q, Chopp M, Bodzin G, Chen H: Temperature modulation of cerebral depolarization during focal cerebral ischemia in rats: Correlation with ischemic injury. J Cereb Blood Flow Metab 1993;13:389–394.
94 Ginsberg MD: The concept of the therapeutic window: A synthesis of critical issues; in Moskowitz MA, Caplan LR (eds): Cerebrovascular Diseases – Nineteenth Princeton Stroke Conference. Boston, Butterworth-Heinemann, 1995, pp 331–351.

95 Ridenour TR, Warner DS, Todd MM, McAllister AC: Mild hypothermia reduces infarct size resulting from temporary but not permanent focal ischemia in rats. Stroke 1992;23:733–738.
96 Xue D, Huang Z-G, Smith KE, Buchan AM: Immediate or delayed mild hypothermia prevents focal cerebral infarction. Brain Res 1992;587:66–72.
97 Chen H, Chopp M, Zhang ZG, Garcia JH: The effect of hypothermia on transient middle cerebral artery occlusion in the rat. J Cereb Blood Flow Metab 1992;12:621–628.
98 Baker CJ, Onesti ST, Solomon RA: Reduction by delayed hypothermia of cerebral infarction following middle cerebral artery occlusion in the rat: A time-course study. J Neurosurg 1992;77:438–444.
99 Kader A, Brisman MH, Maraire N, Huh J-T, Solomon RA: The effect of mild hypothermia on permanent focal ischemia in the rat. Neurosurgery 1992;31:1056–1061.
100 Moyer DJ, Welsh FA, Zager EL: Spontaneous cerebral hypothermia diminishes focal infarction in rat brain. Stroke 1992;23:1812–1816.
101 Zhang R-L, Chopp M, Chen H, Garcia JH, Zhang ZG: Postischemic (1 hour) hypothermia significantly reduces ischemic cell damage in rats subjected to 2 hours of middle cerebral artery occlusion. Stroke 1993;24:1235–1240.
102 Goto Y, Kassell NF, Hiramatsu K, Soleau SW, Lee KS: Effects of intraischemic hypothermia on cerebral damage in a model of reversible focal ischemia. Neurosurgery 1993;32:980–985.
103 Zhang ZG, Chopp M, Chen H: Duration dependent post-ischemic hypothermia alleviates cortical damage after transient middle cerebral artery occlusion in the rat. J Neurol Sci 1993;117:240–244.
104 Karibe H, Chen J, Zarow GJ, Graham SH, Weinstein PR: Delayed induction of mild hypothermia to reduce infarct volume after temporary middle cerebral artery occlusion in rats. J Neurosurg 1994;80:112–119.
105 Markarian GZ, Lee JH, Stein DJ, Hong S-C: Mild hypothermia: Therapeutic window after experimental cerebral ischemia. Neurosurgery 1996;38:542–551.
106 Clifton GL, Jiang JY, Lyeth BG, Jenkins LW, Hamm RJ, Hayes RL: Marked protection by moderate hypothermia after experimental traumatic brain injury. J Cereb Blood Flow Metab 1991;11:114–121.
107 Dietrich WD, Alonso O, Busto R, Globus MY-T, Ginsberg MD: Post-traumatic brain hypothermia reduces histopathological damage following concussive brain injury in the rat. Acta Neuropathol 1994;87:250–258.
108 Bramlett H, Green EJ, Dietrich WD, Busto R, Globus MY-T, Ginsberg MD: Posttraumatic brain hypothermia provides protection from sensorimotor and cognitive behavior deficits. J Neurotrauma 1995;12:289–298.
109 Goss JR, Styren SD, Miller PD, Kochanek PM, Palmer AM, Marion DW, DeKosky ST: Hypothermia attenuates the normal increase in interleukin-1-beta RNA and nerve growth factor following traumatic brain injury in the rat. J Neurotrauma 1995;12:159–167.
110 Marion DW, Obrist WD, Carlier PM, Penrod LE, Darby JM: The use of moderate therapeutic hypothermia for patients with severe head injuries: A preliminary report. J Neurosurg 1993;79:354–362.
111 Clifton GL, Allen S, Barrodale P, Plenger P, Berry J, Koch S, Fletcher J, et al: A phase II study of moderate hypothermia in severe brain injury. J Neurotrauma 1993;10:263–271.
112 Mellergard P, Nordström C-H: Intracerebral temperature in neurosurgical patients. Neurosurgery 1991;28:709–713.
113 Sternau L, Thompson C, Dietrich WD, Busto R, Globus MY-T, Ginsberg MD: Intracranial temperature – Observations in the human brain. J Cereb Blood Flow Metab 1991;11(suppl 2):S123.
114 Marsala M, Vanicky I, Yaksh TL: Effect of graded hypothermia (27 to 34 °C) on behavioral function, histopathology, and spinal blood flow after spinal ischemia in rat. Stroke 1994;25:2038–2046.
115 Yager J, Towfighi J, Vannucci RC: Influence of mild hypothermia on hypoxic-ischemic brain damage in the immature rat. Pediatr Res 1993;34:525–529.
116 Bruno VMG, Goldberg MP, Dugan LL, Giffard RG, Choi DW: Neuroprotective effect of hypothermia in cortical cultures exposed to oxygen-glucose deprivation or excitatory amino acids. J Neurochem 1994;63:1398–1406.

117 Dietrich WD, Busto R, Valdés I, Loor Y: Effects of normothermic versus mild hyperthermic forebrain ischemia in rats. Stroke 1990;21:1318–1325.
118 Kuroiwa T, Bonnekoh P, Hossmann K-A: Prevention of postischemic hyperthermia prevents ischemic injury of CA_1 neurons in gerbils. J Cereb Blood Flow Metab 1990;10:550–556.
119 Sternau LL, Globus MY-T, Dietrich WD, Martinez E, Busto R, Ginsberg MD: Ischemia-induced neurotransmitter release: Effects of mild intraischemic hyperthermia; in Globus MY-T, Dietrich WD (eds): The Role of Neurotransmitters in Brain Injury. New York, Plenum Press, 1992, pp 33–38.
120 Takagi K, Ginsberg MD, Globus MY-T, Martinez E, Busto R: Effect of hyperthermia on glutamate release in ischemic penumbra after middle cerebral artery occlusion in rats occlusion in rats. Am J Physiol 1994;266:H1770–H1776.
121 Dietrich WD, Busto R, Halley M, Valdes I: The importance of brain temperature in alterations of the blood-brain barrier following cerebral ischemia. J Neuropathol Exp Neurol 1990;49:486–497.
122 Dietrich WD, Halley M, Valdés I, Busto R: Interrelationships between increased vascular permeability and acute neuronal damage following temperature-controlled brain ischemia in rats. Acta Neuropathol 1991;81:615–625.
123 Kim Y, Busto R, Dietrich WD, Kraydieh S, Ginsberg MD: Delayed postischemic hyperthermia in awake rats worsens the histopathological outcome of transient focal cerebral ischemia. Stroke 1996;27:2274–2281.
124 Baena RC, Busto R, Dietrich WD, Globus MY-T, Ginsberg MD: Hyperthermia delayed by 24 hours aggravates neuronal damage in rat hippocampus following global ischemia. Neurology 1997;48:768–773.
125 Cook DJ, Orszulak TA, Daly RC, Buda DA: Cerebral hyperthermia during cardiopulmonary bypass in adults. J Thorac Cardiovasc Surg 1996;111:268–269.
126 Maher J, Hachinski V: Hypothermia as a potential treatment for cerebral ischemia. Cerebrovasc Brain Metab Rev 1993;5:277–300.
127 Reith J, Jorgensen HS, Pedersen PM, Nakayama H, Raaschou HO, Jeppesen LL, Olsen TS: Body temperature in acute stroke: Relation to stroke severity, infarct size, mortality, and outcome. Lancet 1996;347:422–425.
128 Meden P, Overgaard K, Pedersen H, Boysen G: The influence of body temperature on infarct volume and thrombolytic therapy in a rat embolic stroke model. Brain Res 1994;647:131–138.

Myron D. Ginsberg, MD, Department of Neurology (D4-5), University of Miami School of Medicine, PO Box 016960, Miami, FL 33101 (USA)

Hsu CY (ed): Ischemic Stroke: From Basic Mechanisms to New Drug Development.
Monogr Clin Neurosci. Basel, Karger, 1998, vol 16, pp 89–115

Apoptosis

Matthew D. Linnik

CNS Molecular Biology, Hoechst Marion Roussel, Inc., and
Department of Neurosurgery, University of Cincinnati College of Medicine,
Cincinnati, Ohio, USA

The Biology of Cell Death

The interruption of cerebral perfusion during a stroke initiates a cascade of detrimental changes in the extracellular compartment of the brain, many of which are the subject of chapters in this volume. In the face of such stresses, an individual cell might respond in one of three ways.

First, a cell could initiate a defensive response that includes, but is not limited to, the up-regulation of defensive genes and proteins, the protective modification of receptors and ion channels, and alterations in organelles designed to buffer changes in the intracellular environment. Second, the cell may have a limited capacity to initiate a defensive response to the ischemic environment. In either of these first two cases, the survival of the cell is primarily dependent on the magnitude and duration of the ischemic insult. Third, it is possible that a cell might respond to the changes in the extracellular environment by activating intracellular mechanisms designed to delete the cell in a suicide-like manner.

A process of autodeletion has been described in many systems as apoptosis or programmed cell death. The definition of these terms was originally highly specific, with apoptosis referring to a morphological cell death distinct from necrosis, while programmed cell death referred to the physiologically appropriate deletion of cells during development and metamorphosis.

The use of the terms apoptosis and programmed cell death remains controversial in ischemia. However, it has recently become clear that there is a biology of cell death associated with ischemia that can be quantitatively described in terms of transcriptional regulation, enzyme activation, and the balance between pro-apoptotic and anti-apoptotic components in a cell. Furthermore, this cell death biology appears to involve a cascade of events leading up to a point where a cell becomes irreversibly committed to die. While these investigations are still early, this chapter will describe the observations that have led to an appreciation of the role of cell death biology in ischemia and suggest where future experiments are likely to lead to additional understanding of the pathophysiology of acute neurodegenerative disorders.

Why Might Neurons Commit Suicide?

It is not immediately obvious why a postmitotic, nonreplicating neuron would consider autodeletion in a stroke since there is no chance for that neuron to be replaced. However, it is important to appreciate that each neuron retains the capacity for programmed cell death that was necessary for prenatal neuronal modelling. During brain development, almost half of all progenitor neurons are deleted in the process of developing appropriate neuronal circuits, often because the developing neuron fails to acquire adequate growth factors from the target tissue [1, 2]. This cell death program is repressed in the surviving neurons by mechanisms that are poorly understood and ideally remains repressed for the life span of the organism.

Why might a brain cell activate components of this latent suicide program following an ischemic insult? While specific data is limited, one reasonable explanation for the activation of a cell death program is that the deletion of a single cell is an altruistic event, designed to prevent large-scale inflammation and the disastrous consequences of mutation and transformation into a proliferative phenotype.

One of the basic tenants of apoptosis is that the cell death occurs in the absence of significant lymphocyte infiltration and inflammation. This permits the deletion of specific cells without additional cell loss in the surrounding tissue due to inflammation-induced necrosis. While it is clear that there is inflammatory cell infiltration in cerebral ischemia, there is also a component of necrosis that accompanies the core of the infarction where cell death is primarily due to metabolic failure. This lymphocyte infiltration is not apparent until 6 h in reperfusion models and 12 h in permanent occlusion models, reaching a peak at 5 days postischemia [3–7].

An autodeletion response also makes sense if one considers the detrimental consequences of DNA mutations and the potential transformation of a neuron or glial cell into a rapidly replicating, autonomous tissue mass. In almost all cases, it is preferable to sacrifice a selected area of tissue, rather than risk genomic mutations. Consistent with this hypothesis is the activation of p53 transcription following ischemia [8, 9]. The normal function of p53 is to delay cell division and permit repair of DNA damage prior to undergoing a replicative cycle. p53 also has a critical function in the execution of apoptosis when the DNA damage is too extensive.

Two Key Determinants of Cell Death: Transcription and Enzyme Activation

The primary mechanisms that regulate life and death decisions in apoptosis can be roughly divided into two categories. The first category is enzyme-based and consists primarily of the endonucleases, interleukin (IL)-1β converting enzyme (ICE) family of proteases and the calcium-activated neutral proteinases or calpains [10]. The key experimental questions related to the enzymes concern the mechanisms of activation and the identification of critical substrates.

The second category of investigation in apoptosis concerns transcriptional mediated components and consists primarily of the bcl-2 family of proteins, the tumor suppressors (i.e. p53), and a variety of transcription factors. The basic description of these mechanisms and the cell biology associated with the expression or deletion of these components occupy a large body of data in this area.

While both of these areas will be discussed in detail, they will be discussed independently as a matter of necessity. A major unresolved dilemma in the field of cell death biology concerns the integration of these two areas that independently appear to dramatically influence survival decisions in the cell.

Finally, it should be mentioned that a third area of research is evolving that relates to the signal transduction cascades that regulate apoptosis [11]. However, the neuron-specific research efforts in this area are embryonic and they will not be considered in detail.

Apoptosis-Related Enzymes in Stroke

A molecular analysis of cell death mechanisms clearly indicates that neurons are capable of autodeletion. It also appears that much of the critical machinery for cell death is constitutively present in neurons, awaiting appropriate signals for activation. Some of this cell death machinery takes the form of enzymes that are constitutively expressed in a pro-form or inactive form. The activation signals are not well understood, but the consequences of activation include the degradation of key structural, regulatory and genomic elements, including the DNA, the cell cytoskeleton, and regulatory proteins necessary for maintenance of cellular homeostasis.

Endonucleases Distinguish Apoptosis from Necrosis

A distinguishing feature of apoptosis is the activation of a calcium-dependent endonuclease and the subsequent degradation of DNA into oligonucleosomal fragments. This type of cleavage is typically established by gel electrophoresis where size fractionation of the DNA results in an oligonucleosomal ladder pattern reflecting multimers of nucleosomes which are approximately 180–200 bases in length.

The reason oligonucleosomal ladders are used to distinguish between apoptosis and necrosis is best understood by considering the secondary and tertiary structure of DNA. The double helical nature of DNA permits both single-stranded breaks, for which many elegant repair mechanisms exist, and double-stranded breaks which are much more disruptive and which cannot be easily repaired.

Lysosomes are normally isolated from the cell in vesicles and are released in necrosis where they are free to attack the DNA. Lysosomes are crude instruments for the cleavage of DNA, and typically produce many more single-stranded breaks than double-stranded breaks. In contrast, endonucleases are specialized for double-stranded cleavage where they produce exclusively double-stranded breaks in the DNA.

The reason for the regular repeating pattern of 200 bases monomers involves the accessibility of the DNA to the endonucleases. Because of the high negative charge on the phosphodiester backbone, histones have evolved to assist in the dense packing of the DNA into a beaded structure. The smallest subunit of this structure consists of three loops of DNA wound around an octamer of histones, occupying approximate 200 bases of DNA. These nucleosomes are relatively inaccessible to the endonuclease, while the internucleosomal regions are not complexed to histones and are readily accessible to the endonuclease. Thus, the activated endonucleases initially attack the DNA at the internucleosomal regions which are the most readily accessible regions.

Apoptotic DNA Cleavage Is a Prominent Feature in Ischemia

There is a great deal of evidence that apoptotic DNA fragmentation is a prominent feature in ischemic cell death and the importance of this fragmentation has been noted [12]. Electrophoretic evidence of endonuclease-mediated fragmentation can be observed after focal ischemia [13–16] and global ischemia [17–22].

An interesting series of studies by MacManus et al. [21] has shown that ischemia-induced DNA fragmentation is not a random necrotic event, but an ordered and deliberate destruction of genomic DNA that is consistent with an apoptotic death. These investigators compared DNA fragmentation patterns in neocortex, hippocampus, and striatum following occlusion/reperfusion with DNA integrity after decapitation. The DNA fragmentation appeared as an ordered, oligonucleosomal pattern in the ischemic animals, while random fragmentation with no apparent higher order structure was observed in DNA extracted from decapitated tissue.

Two aspects of the DNA fragmentation studies point to the importance of apoptosis as a potentially critical contributor to the early pathogenesis of ischemic neuronal death. First, several studies have demonstrated that the initiation of DNA fragmentation occurs early in the cell death cascade and precedes the appearance of morphological changes in the cells [15, 16, 19, 20]. Second, in the focal ischemia models, the DNA fragmentation appears to concentrate in the pharmacological penumbra, i.e., those cells that are potentially amenable to pharmacological intervention. Apoptotic cells accumulate along the inner margin of the infarction and appear to expand with the ischemic lesion, while necrotic cells are predominantly found in the ischemic core [15, 16, 23–25].

The initial appearance of DNA fragmentation in focal ischemia occurs within 0.5–1 h after the occlusion [15, 16]. This precedes the appearance of morphological changes in cells which become evident by light microscopy beginning 4 h after the initiation of ischemia. DNA end-labeling methods [26] have been used to establish that the maximum number of fragmentation-positive apoptotic cells occurs 24–48 h after focal ischemia [15, 16, 25].

Similar findings have also been observed in global ischemia, although the time course for all events including cell death is delayed. As in focal ischemia, the fragmentation in global ischemia is mediated by endonucleases [17–19] and initially precedes the appearance of morphological neurodegeneration in the sensitive CA1 region of the hippocampus [20].

Most of the approaches described above depend on extensive, double-stranded DNA fragmentation. However, there are no mechanisms for a cell to repair its DNA when it is digested in a double-stranded fashion into relatively large fragments. Furthermore, the 180–300 base fragments that typically resolved on a DNA ladder gel represent far more genomic destruction than is necessary to delete a cell. Recent studies indicate that digestion of the genome in apoptotic cells occurs in a stepwise fashion, with the initial appearance of 300-kb bands, followed by 50-kb bands and subsequent destruction into smaller, oligonucleosomal fragments [27–29]. This initial digestion is sufficient to cause the chromatin condensation associated with apoptotic nuclear morphology.

The DNA degradation in reversible focal ischemia also proceeds in this stepwise fashion. Using pulsed field methodology, Charriaut-Marlangue et al. [30] demonstrated the degradation of cerebral cortex DNA into 300-kb fragments, followed by further digestion to 50-kb fragments and finally smaller oligonucleosomal fragments. The 300-kb fragments were maximal at 6 h post-ischemia (the first time point measured) and were declining by 18 h as the smaller fragments began to predominate. Although it seems likely that the same cells that exhibit the large, initial digestion products go on to produce oligonucleosomal fragments, this point remains to be proven.

What Percent of Ischemic Cell Death Is Apoptotic?

A difficult question concerns the absolute number of apoptotic cells and the relative percentage of cell death that can be attributed to apoptosis relative to necrosis. Apoptotic cells in other systems are notorious for the rate at which they are rapidly cleared from the tissue. This rapid rate of clearance involves a basic tenant of apoptosis, namely that apoptotic cell death occurs in the absence of inflammatory cell infiltration. The mechanism for this clearance may involve the appearance of cell surface signals, possibly phosphatidylserine residues [31, 32], and the recruitment of neighboring cells to assist in the engulfment of apoptotic cells. To date, no one has reported on the rate at which apoptotic cells are cleared in the ischemic cortex. Furthermore, it seems likely that the rate of clearance of apoptotic neurons in ischemia could vary during the maturation of the lesion, as more and more cells are dying and therefore become incapable deleting neighboring cells.

The importance of determining the rate of disappearance of apoptotic cells in the CNS is of more than academic interest as it influences one's ability to interpret the magnitude of changes observed in biochemical and molecular analyses of the ischemic regions. For example, if one were to determine the rate of activation of a pro-apoptotic enzyme in the ischemic region, the net effect of this activation would be influenced by the number of apoptotic cells present in the tissue at that time. If apoptotic cells were rapidly cleared, even large changes in an enzyme activity might be masked by the rapid clearance and subsequent deletion of those cells. Thus, the magnitude of any pro-apoptotic change in a tissue is based on both the rate of appearance or activation of that observation minus the rate of clearance of those cells.

A definitive calculation of the percent of ischemic death relative to necrotic death would also be heavily influenced by the outcome measures associated with the particular experimental design. One might expect to arrive at very different conclusions depending on whether one were measuring morphology, electrophoretic DNA fragmentation, TUNEL staining, or a pharmacological response. Obviously, the choice of model (global or focal), the nature of the infarctions (permanent or reperfusion) and even the species and strain of animal would have an impact on this analysis.

The relative contributions of apoptosis and necrosis to ischemic cell death may not be fully resolved for several years. However, this knowledge could be very important for predicting the optimal therapeutic interventions, the time constraints associated with a specific intervention relative to the onset of the ischemia, and possibly help determine if cells communicate death signals to neighboring neurons in ischemia.

Protease Activation during Apoptosis

The endonucleases are only one component of the enzymatic machinery that is activated during apoptosis. There is now increasing evidence that proteases play a key role in the cell death process. In several experimental models, including cell-free systems and enucleated cells, proteolysis often appears to be a dominant regulator of cell death. Furthermore, some of these proteases have proven amenable to pharmacological manipulation and exhibit neuroprotective effects in experimental stroke, suggesting that this may be a very important area for continued investigation.

The ICE Family of Proteases

Several proteases have now been implicated in apoptosis, although most have not been systematically investigated in cerebral ischemic models. The greater apoptosis scientific community now considers the proteins of the ICE/ced-3 family to be the most important and highly conserved members of the apoptotic proteases. These enzymes were initially described in the nematode *Caenorhabditis elegans*, as the cell death executioner, ced-3. Subsequently, ced-3 was shown to have significant homology to the human enzyme, ICE [33]. This protease converts inactive pro-IL-1 to active IL-1 by cleavage after a highly conserved aspartate residue [34]. Ectopic expression of ICE can independently induce apoptosis in serveral cell types, including neurons [35].

The name ICE was coined because of the high degree of substrate specificity that had been determined for this enzyme. However, it is now clear that ICE can induce apoptosis in cells that do not express pro-IL-1, and an intensive search is underway to identify other substrates for this enzyme. In addition, several homologs of ICE have now been identified as cysteine proteases that can also function in cell death pathways.

Currently, very little is known about the role of the ced-3/ICE family of proteases in cerebral ischemia. Several investigations into the role of cytokines during the postischemic period have revealed that IL-1 mRNA levels are dramatically increased after ischemia [36–39]. The increase in IL-1 mRNA may be important because ischemia causes a reduction in transcription of new mRNA. Thus, the IL-1 mRNA increases during a time when most housekeeping genes are being down-regulated. However, the functional significance of this observation has not been established since it is currently unknown if this increase in mRNA translates into an increase in pro-IL-1 protein. Pro-IL-1 must then be enzymatically processed by ICE to be activated and it is currently unknown if ICE or an ICE homolog is active and available to generate active cytokine.

There are examples of apoptosis models that require activation of an ICE-like enzyme, but do not require pro-IL-1 expression or processing. However, there is now evidence that the processing of IL-1 can contribute to cell death in a manner analogous to the pharmacological potentiation of cell death. This pharmacological potentiation of apoptosis by IL-1 may contribute to ischemic neuronal death, since blockade of the IL-1 receptor can reduce infarct volume.

Betz et al. [40] used an adenoviral vector to increase the expression of the endogenous IL-1 receptor antagonist in cerebral spinal fluid and observed a neuroprotective effect from this treatment. Similar results were reported when IL-1 was blocked by zinc protoporphyrin or an anti-IL-1β antibody [41]. In this study, both infarct volume and edema were attenuated by inhibition of IL-1β. More recently, Friedlander et al. [42] have evaluated transgenic mice that overexpress the IL-1 receptor antagonist and observed that these animals produce smaller infarctions and have a better neurological outcome relative to their nontransgenic littermates when challenged by unilateral permanent middle cerebral artery occlusion. In all of these studies, it is believed that the observed protection is due to an attenuation of secreted extracellular IL-1β, rather than any effect on the ICE-like protease. This is normally considered to be an inflammatory component of the postischemic sequelae, although it is quite possible that the inflammation and the apoptosis might be interrelated.

These results clearly indicate that IL-1 production is detrimental in stroke. However, it is unclear if the IL-1 production is related to lymphocyte infiltration or endogenous production in resident cortical cells. Furthermore, the magnitude of increase in active IL-1 protein levels after a stroke has not been established, and it remains unclear if the detrimental effects of cytokine production are directly related to ICE-like protease activation and apoptosis or are independently related to inflammatory cell activation. An obvious important issue will be to resolve which of the ICE-like proteases are activated by ischemia, and then to determine if the activated protease(s) can process pro-IL-1 into an active form. It will also be important to determine if the source of the pro-IL-1 and ICE is the resident astrocytes, neurons, and glia, or whether the increases in IL-1 depend on lymphocyte infiltration as this will influence the mechanisms one can consider for intervention.

The ICE/ced-3 family of proteases will likely attract a great deal of attention in the near future. Recent observations from cell culture systems suggest that inhibition of this family of proteases can dramatically inhibit cell death [43, 44]. This inhibition of apoptosis occurs in a manner that is completely consistent with the observations in the nematodes where ced-3 is essential and obligatory for developmental cell death. Evolution has made this system a great deal more complex in mammals than it is in nematodes, and there is an expanding list of family members [45, 46].

Several biochemical and molecular issues related to the activation and function of ICE/ced-3 proteases remain unresolved. Perhaps most importantly is the very poor understanding of the factors that are necessary to process the inactive pro-enzymes to the active enzyme. The X-ray crystal structure of ICE has been solved and indicates that the active enzyme consists of a tetramer containing two copies each of the p20 and p10 subunits [47]. Therefore, the pro-enzyme must have some processing mechanism that cleaves these domains from the pro-enzyme and permits assembly of the active configuration. The ICE family members also share homology regarding pro-enzyme structure and active site domains, yet they often have different substrate specificity. It is likely that these proteases can act on several substrates, and there is a great deal of interest in understanding which substrates are most important in the cell death process.

The Calpain Family of Cysteine Proteinases

While the ICE-like proteases have captured the greatest attention in the apoptosis community, a less glamorous but therapeutically relevant family of proteases known as the calcium-activated neutral proteinases, or calpains, have been strongly implicated in both apoptosis and ischemia.

The calpains are a family of homologous proteins that differ by their tissue distribution and sensitivity to calcium. They are most easily classified into three classes depending on whether they are activated by low micromolar levels of calcium (μ-calpain or calpain I), high micromolar levels of calcium (m-calpain or calpain II), and a more recently described intermediate form (μ/m-calpain) [48, 49]. Tissue-specific isoforms have also been described for stomach and skeletal muscle, but the significance of these isoforms is only beginning to be appreciated [50].

All calpains are structurally similar, and are composed of two subunits, an 80-kD large subunit and a 29-kD small subunit. Each subunit contains similar calmodulin-like EF hand regions for calcium binding, while only the large subunit contains the catalytic domain (domain II) that shares homology with other cysteine proteinases [51].

While the exact regulation of calpain is not well understood, it is believed that calcium binding to the EF hand regions provides a two key conformational changes in the protein. The first change is an autolytic cleavage of domain I from the pro-protein. The autolysis of the 80-kD precursor protein to a 76-kD activated isoform has been used to distinguish areas of activated calpain in the brain [52]. The calcium binding is also thought to release the catalytic domain (domain II) from an inhibitory interaction with domain III by virtue of a flip-flop mechanism that permits full activation of the protease.

Role of Calpain in Apoptosis and Ischemia

The calpains are ideally positioned to contribute to cell death in neurons. First these enzymes are constitutively expressed as inactive pro-enzymes, and are activated by high calcium levels. Second, they are not digestive enzymes, as they seem to alter substrates rather than destroy substrates. The implication of this limited proteolysis is that calpain seems to serve a signaling function, as in the case of protein kinase C, where limited proteolysis by calpain activates the kinase domain [53].

μ-Calpain activation has been causally implicated in several lymphocyte apoptosis models, including dexamethasone treatment, low-level irradiation, and macromolecular synthesis inhibition [54–56]. However, it is also clear that calpain is not involved in all apoptotic cell deaths. For example, calpain inhibitors are not effective in NGF-deprived neuronal cultures [57, 58] or in low $K+$ induced apoptosis of cerebellar granule neurons [59], or in selected types of lymphocyte apoptosis [60]. Thus, calpain illustrates what appears to be an emerging theme in apoptosis, namely that differentiated cells can employ a variety of signal transduction mechanisms to activate and execute a cell suicide process.

While the role and function of calpain in classical apoptosis models continues to be evaluated, there is a growing body of evidence that the calpains are present in neurons, are activated by ischemia, and that calpain activation contributes to neuronal death. It has long been recognized that excitotoxicity activates μ-calpain and induces structural protein breakdown in vitro and in vivo [61, 62]. In focal cerebral ischemia, the calpain-specific breakdown of the structural protein spectrin (or fodrin) precedes the appearance of morphologically defined neurodegeneration by several hours in both cortex and striatum [63, 64]. The increase in calpain-mediated proteolysis occurs in a biphasic manner in the peri-infarct region, with the initial appearance of spectrin fragments appearing within 1–2 h of the ischemic insult. A second phase of larger magnitude develops between 6 and 24 h that coincides with the tissue that will ultimately infarct [65].

The time difference between the onset of calpain-specific proteolysis and morphological appearance of neurodegeneration is more pronounced in global ischemia than in focal ischemia, and it has been suggested that calpain-mediated proteolysis in hippocampus occurs in three phases [66, 67]. Ten minutes of global ischemia is sufficient to produce the initial appearance of spectrin degradation, a predegeneration phase, which initiates within 15 min and lasts up to 4 h. A second predegeneration phase develops between 12 and 24 h in the CA1 region, while a postdegeneration phase accompanies the morphological appearance of degeneration in the hippocampus. Interestingly, sublethal ischemia of 3 min induced the first predegeneration phase of spectrin breakdown, but not the second predegeneration phase which appeared to parallel a commitment to cell death.

Pharmacological inhibition of calpain provides significant neuroprotection in global ischemia. This was first demonstrated by Lee et al. [66] who showed that infusion of the calpain inhibitor leupeptin could provide almost complete protection of the hippocampal CA1 neurons in gerbils exposed to 10 min of global ischemia. Similar results have been reported for calpain inhibitor 1 [68]. This therapeutic approach also preserves electrophysiological responses and synaptic transmission, suggesting that these neurons remain functional [66, 69].

The protection observed in global ischemia has also been observed in focal ischemia using a variety of calpain inhibitors. These studies demonstrate that calpain inhibitors attenuate ischemia-induced proteolysis and edema, as well as reduce infarct volume [65]. The protective effects are elicited in a dose-dependent manner, and the compounds continue to provide tissue preservation even when administration is delayed for 3 h from the initiation of ischemia [70, 71]. This notable therapeutic window of opportunity is consistent with the inhibition of the second phase of calpain-mediated proteolysis and supports the hypothesis that this delayed proteolysis contributes to the commitment phase of cell death.

There are several important questions related to calcium binding and calpain activation which are not well understood. For example, it has been difficult to determine the molar ratio of calcium ions required for activation. Interestingly, the amount of calcium required for activation is reduced in the presence of lipid and this has led to the suggestion that the threshold for calpain activation might be reduced near cell membranes. Second, the role of the small subunit is poorly understood and recombinant protein expression studies suggest that the small subunit is not required for activity [72].

Other issues related to the role of calcium in the activation of calpain are also outstanding. For example, one of the first steps in the calcium-induced activation of calpain is autolytic cleavage of domain I. It is not known if this autolysis is necessary for activation of the catalytic component in domain II. In addition, it is not known what role calcium has in the activation-induced autolysis of calpain, which eventually leads to full autolysis and inactivation. Is calcium still required after initial activation, or will transient exposure to high levels of calcium lead to activation and depletion of enzyme, even though calcium levels return to normal? This suggests an interesting mechanism that might contribute to ischemic preconditioning, i.e. that brief transient ischemia activates and subsequently depletes part of the intracellular calpain pool that can only be replaced by transcription and translation of new protein.

Transcription-Based Mechanisms: Effect of Inhibiting Protein Synthesis

An important experiment that can be used to help differentiate apoptosis from necrosis involves examining the role of new protein synthesis in the death of a cell. Protein synthesis is an obvious requirement for all cells and inhibiting protein synthesis for extended periods will be toxic to virtually every cell. However, apoptotic cell death is attenuated by protein synthesis inhibitors in most in vitro models of neuronal apoptosis, including NGF deprivation-induced death of superior cervical ganglia neurons [73], low potassium-induced death of cultured cortical neurons [59], or in selected sublines of PC12 cells following NGF removal [58].

Protein synthesis inhibitors like cycloheximide provide an opportunity to determine if new proteins are synthesized during cell death that actually contribute to the cell death, as would be predicted in an apoptosis model. In contrast, if death is purely necrotic, inhibition of protein synthesis should not improve outcome, and might even worsen outcome due to the inherent toxicity associated with this treatment.

The potentially detrimental role of ischemia-induced gene expression has been assessed by evaluating the effect of protein synthesis inhibitors on CA1 hippocampal neurons after temporary global ischemia. Goto et al. [74] initially reported that systemic administration of a protein synthesis inhibitor could dramatically reduce hippocampal cell death in global ischemia. This observation was subsequently confirmed [75, 76], or refuted [77, 78] using multiple dosing paradigms and several variations of the global ischemia model.

Several possibilities could explain the discrepancies in these observations. However, direct comparisons of these studies is complicated because most did not determine the magnitude and duration of protein synthesis inhibition. In addition, it is not clear which specific, newly transcribed protein(s) are involved in this cycloheximide effect, and the extent to which this translation must be attenuated is currently unknown.

In focal ischemia, protein synthesis inhibitors appear to be an effective mechanism to reduce infarct volume. Using a continuous infusion of cycloheximide directly into the lateral cerebral ventricle, a profound and persistent decrease in protein synthesis was established [13]. This reduction in protein synthesis caused a significant reduction in infarct volume following permanent focal ischemia, suggesting that new protein synthesis might contribute to cell death in a stroke.

These initial studies have been extended in a very interesting direction by Du et al. [79] who examined the effect of cycloheximide on mild, transient focal ischemia. These investigators were able to demonstrate that 30 min of ischemia caused a slowly evolving infarction, an observation reminiscent of the delayed neuronal death observed in hippocampal neurons after brief periods of global ischemia. The time course for the evolution of the infarction in this transient focal model is even more delayed than in global ischemia, with no infarction evident at 1 day, some evolution apparent at 3 days, and a very large infarction (equivalent to 90 min of occlusion) apparent at 14 days.

The effect of cycloheximide in this model of delayed neuronal death is quite dramatic. When the 30-min occlusion was preceded by a single intraperitoneal injection of cycloheximide, the infarction was almost completely abolished out to 14 days after the occlusion. These studies strongly suggest that newly translated proteins play an important role in ischemia-induced death of both neurons and glial cells.

The identity of the important translation products is almost completely undetermined, but several starting points are suggested from in vitro apoptosis models, especially the well-described NGF-deprived superior cervical ganglia model. Several genes are up-regulated in these neurons when the apoptotic cascade is initiated and some of these genes have been documented to be increased following ischemia. For example, increases in c-fos and c-jun expression accompanies chromatin condensation in the ganglia cells [80] and these immediate early genes are induced in cerebral cortex by ischemia [81–83]. Other genes that are induced during neuronal apoptosis in vitro and in ischemia in vivo include junB, and the NGFI genes [80, 84–87].

The fact that many of the ischemia- and apoptosis-induced genes are transcription factors has made it difficult to distinguish between epiphenomena and events that are critical to the cell death cascade. The complexities are not only intellectual but also technical, since one needs methodology to manipulate a specific gene in order to prove functional significance. The technical hurdles can be overcome in vitro by injecting neutralizing antibodies into specific cells and following the progression of that cell [80, 88] but this is not feasible in vivo. The evaluation of specific gene products in vivo is more complex, but successful manipulation has been established with antisense approaches against c-fos [89], transgenic approaches for bcl-2, p53, superoxide dismutase, and nitric oxide synthetase [90–93], and viral vector-mediated gene therapy for IL-1, bcl-2, and the glucose transporter [40, 94–96].

Functional Importance of the Bcl-2/Ced-9 Gene Families

The ced-9/bcl-2 family of proteins are remarkable for their apparently unique ability to inhibit physiological and pathological cell death, including neuronal cell death. These membrane-bound intercellular proteins protect cells from a variety of insults, including several that have been implicated in cerebral ischemia (see below). However, to appreciate the integral role of the bcl-2/ced-9 gene family in apoptosis and cerebral ischemia, it is useful to briefly review the experiments that led to the discovery of these genes.

Bcl-2 was originally identified as a proto-oncogene responsible for certain B-cell follicular lymphomas. In these lymphomas the bcl-2 gene becomes translocated from its normal position on chromosome 18 to band q32 of chromosome 14. This places the bcl-2 gene under the control of the immunoglobulin heavy chain promoter, resulting in overexpression of bcl-2 in these B cells [97, 98]. Interestingly, these t(14;18) B cells retain a relatively normal phenotype, and neoplasia develops as a consequence of the suppression of cell death, rather than the induction of hyperproliferation.

The discovery of the ced-9 gene comes from an entirely independent line of research in the nematode, *C. elegans*. This organism produces 1,090 progenitor cells of which 131 undergo developmental programmed cell death. Mutational studies revealed that ced-9 gain of function mutants suppressed normal programmed cell death, while ced-9 deletions caused inappropriate programmed cell death and embryonic lethality [99]. These two lines of research converged when the ced-9 gene was cloned and peptide sequence and structural homology to bcl-2 was detected. Remarkably, overexpression of the human bcl-2 gene in ced-9 loss-of-function mutants demonstrated that bcl-2 could functionally substitute for ced-9 in *C. elegans*, suggesting conservation of cell survival mechanisms in organisms separated by 600 million years of evolution [100, 101]

Investigations in mammalian cells reveal the bcl-2 can prevent both apoptotic and necrotic death from a wide variety of insults [102–104]. In many of these examples, the cell death stimuli are directly relevant to ischemic pathophysiology, including glutamate [105–107], lipid peroxidation [107–109], hypoxia and anoxia [111, 112], elevated calcium [107].

The endogenous expression of bcl-2 is originally high in the developing brain but progressively declines with aging [113, 114]. Interestingly, hippocampal bcl-2 levels correlate with relative degrees of susceptibility to ischemia. For example, basal bcl-2 immunoreactivity is high in the ischemia-resistant pyramidal neurons of CA3, while it is present in very low levels in the ischemia-sensitive CA1 region. Bcl-2 expression is also high in the brainstem in regions where autonomic function is typically preserved, even during extensive loss of neuronal function [115]. However, bcl-2 staining is relatively selective, and is present in very low levels in certain regions like the cortex.

Ischemia Alters Bcl-2 Expression

The regulation of Bcl-2 expression has recently been evaluated in focal and global ischemia models. Chen et al. [116] assessed the expression of bcl-2 protein following 60 or 120 min of focal cerebral ischemia. They observed that bcl-2 levels increase in the border zone immediately outside the region of the infarction in the animals exposed to 120 min of ischemia. This increase in expression was not confined to neurons as it also increased in sublethally injured glial cells. Sixty minutes of ischemia produced little morphological evidence of damage, and these animals exhibited a widespread increase in bcl-2 immunoreactivity in the frontoparietal cortex.

Sublethal global ischemia induced by bilateral common carotid ligation (2 min) produced an increase in bcl-2 immunoreactivity in CA1 neurons by 24 h that persisted for 4 days after the ischemia [117]. In contrast, extending the period of ischemia to a lethal 5 min caused a decrease in bcl-2 levels that paralleled the morphological degradation of the neurons. Interestingly, the sublethal ischemia that induced bcl-2 was also sufficient to induce tolerance to a secondary 5-min ischemic challenge, suggesting a potential role for bcl-2 in the acquisition of resistance to delayed neuronal death.

A consistent induction of bcl-2 in surviving neurons was not observed in hippocampus following global ischemia induced by cardiac stun, although a transient increase in some surviving neurons was suggested [115]. However, bcl-2 levels uniformly decreased in neurons with morphological evidence of degeneration, in a manner similar to that observed with 5 min bilateral carotid ligation. These combined studies are consistent with the hypothesis that bcl-2 may be induced by sublethal injury, but is diminished in neurons that are irreversibly committed to die. The results are also consistent with the possibility that bcl-2 expression influences cell survival in ischemia, particularly along the border zone of the infarction.

Pro-Apoptotic and Anti-Apoptotic Members of the Bcl-2 Family

To fully appreciate the role of the bcl-2 gene family in neuronal pathophysiology, one must recognize that the original ced-9 gene in *C. elegans* has evolved many members in the bcl-2 family [118, 119]. All bcl-2 family members described to date have a role in regulating survival decisions in the cell, but not all members prevent apoptosis as some members actually can enhance cell death. These family members compete with each other by mechanisms that are thought to involve protein-protein interactions. The preferred configuration of the bcl-2 family is as dimers, and highly conserved BH1 and BH2 domains regulate this dimerization [120–122]. Ultimately, it is the balance between pro-apoptotic and anti-apoptotic family members, and their associated dimerization partners, that is thought to determine the fate of a cell from a bcl-2 perspective.

Bcl-X is an anti-apoptotic family member that has a much wider distribution than bcl-2 and is present in many neurons [115, 123, 124]. Bax is another family member that is widely distributed like bcl-X, but has the opposite function as it promotes cell death [125]. The regulation of these family members has recently been investigated in a model of global cerebral ischemia.

The same experiments that reported a down-regulation of bcl-2 in dying neurons also observed an up-regulation of the pro-apoptotic bax protein in neurons with morphological evidence of degeneration [115]. These findings are also consistent with the hypothesis that differential expression of bcl-2 family members influences the sensitivity of specific neurons to ischemia and may actively participate in the cell death cascade.

Therapeutic Manipulation of Bcl-2 Expression

Several investigators have tried to take advantage of properties of bcl-2 by selectively overexpressing the protein in the brain. This expression can be enhanced by transgenic overexpression or by viral gene transfer. To determine the effect of bcl-2 expression on ischemic neuronal survival in vivo, viable transgenic mice were developed that overexpressed bcl-2 in the brain [90]. These animals exhibited hypertrophy in many regions of the nervous system, possibly due to bcl-2-mediated inhibition of normal developmental programmed cell death.

The transgenic bcl-2 overexpressing animals were subjected to permanent middle cerebral artery occlusion to evaluate the effect of this genetic modification on cell survival. The volume of brain infarction in the transgenic mice was reduced by 50% as compared with wild-type mice. The interpretation of these experiments is complicated by the hypertrophic brains in transgenic animals and the lack of comparative cerebrovascular physiology between the transgenic and the wild-type controls. However, the results certainly suggest that bcl-2 can influence cell survival after an ischemic challenge.

Localized increases in bcl-2 expression have also been generated by injecting viral expression vectors containing the bcl-2 gene directly into the brain parenchyma. A replication-defective herpes simplex virus containing human bcl-2 under the regulatory control of the HSV I/E 4/5 promoter was directly injected in the cerebral cortex parenchyma to obtain site-selective overexpression of bcl-2 [94]. A control group was also injected with identical vectors that substituted the β-galactosidase gene for the bcl-2 gene. The HSV-bcl-2-injected animals displayed elevated levels of bcl-2 immunoreactivity in the area surrounding the injection site. They also displayed localized neuroprotection in the area around the injection site relative to the animals injected with the HSV-β-galactosidase vector.

A similar approach was also adopted using a bicistronic vector capable of expressing both bcl-2 and β-galactosidase in the same cell [95]. In these experiments, the virus was injected into the striatum, animals were exposed to 1 h ischemia, and the number of β-galactosidase-positive cells was counted at 48 h as an index of the efficacy of the bcl-2. While the combined bcl-2/β-galactosidase vector did not produce a decrease in total damage to the striatum, there was an increase in the number of β-galactosidase-positive neurons, indicating that neurons which expressed bcl-2 were relatively spared from the effects of the ischemia.

The mechanism by which bcl-2 provides this protection is not fully understood and is currently comprised of two lines of evidence. First, bcl-2 seems to function in an antioxidant pathway to prevent apoptosis [108, 109, 111]. The protein has a single transmembrane region that localizes it primarily to mitochondrial and nuclear membranes and it is at these sites where the anti-apoptotic and antioxidant effects are observed [112, 126–128]. However, there are reports that bcl-2 can inhibit apoptosis at very low oxygen tension [110] suggesting that reactive oxygen species are not involved in bcl-2-mediated protection. Furthermore, bcl-2 can block apoptosis in cells that lack mitochondrial DNA and therefore do not have a functional respiratory chain, suggesting that neither apoptosis nor the protective effect of bcl-2 depends on mitochondrial respiration [129]. Currently, this line of investigation is generating much debate, and likely will require additional investigation before resolution.

The other mechanism involves the relative expression and dimerization of the pro-apoptotic and anti-apoptotic bcl-2 family members [118, 119]. Oltvai et al. [125] first proposed that the anti-apoptotic action of bcl-2 depended on dimerization with bax, and that overexpression of bax could counter the effect of bcl-2 and accelerate cell death [120]. This theme is consistent with the description of the long and short forms of bcl-x (bcl-xl and bcl-xs, respectively) where bcl-xl mimics the protective effect of bcl-2, but the bcl-xs acts as a functional antagonist of both bcl-2 and bcl-xl [111, 123]. Exceptions to these dimerization rules have been described [130] suggesting that additional experiments will be necessary to resolve these controversies. However, the need to resolve the mechanisms from a cell biology perspective does not diminish the fact that several lines of evidence suggest that appropriate manipulation of the bcl-2 family may have therapeutic benefit in ischemia.

Role of the Tumor Suppressor p53 in Stroke

p53 is a tumor suppressor protein by virtue of its ability to interrupt the cell cycle and induce apoptosis [131–133]. p53 protein expression is dramatically up-regulated during cell injury, including excitotoxicity, and has been shown to be associated with neuronal apoptosis in vivo [134, 135].

The expression of p53 is up-regulated by ischemia and may be involved in regulating cell survival. Chopp and co-workers [8, 9] followed the time course of p53 expression after a stroke and observed that p53 levels increased in cells destined to die. The functional significance of this change in expression is strongly supported by ischemia experiments conducted in transgenic p53 null mutants. Animals lacking the p53 gene exhibited a reduction in infarct volume when compared to wild-type controls [91]. Similarly, transgenic p53 null mutants were also protected from kainate-induced cell death [136], suggesting that p53 may play a critical role in the excitotoxic component of cell death.

The exact mechanism by which p53 expression influences cell survival in ischemia, or whether it interacts with apoptotic proteases and the bcl-2 family, is not well understood. On the surface, it would not seem that the antiproliferative effects of p53 associated with cell cycle regulation would have an important role in ischemia. However, the cell cycle-related protein cyclin D1 is up-regulated in in vitro apoptosis models, and appears to play a critical role in establishing the fate of the cell [88]. As for interactions with other apoptosis components, it is clear that anti-apoptotic members of the bcl-2 family can inhibit p53-mediated apoptosis, but the link between these systems has not been fully elucidated and it has not been established if this is functional in the nervous system [137, 138].

The Morphology of Apoptosis

The term apoptosis was derived from morphological observations that sought to distinguish two clearly distinct forms of cell death. Necrotic death is considered a passive death that involves a failure of cellular homeostasis. Typical components of a necrotic death include a loss of membrane integrity, a failure of mitochondrial function and associated loss of ATP production, and a failure to maintain ionic homeostasis. Cells and mitochondria typically swell during necrotic death due to the influx of water. Intracellular membranes fragment and there is a loss of cytoplasmic integrity, although the nucleus and chromatin may remain intact until relatively late in the process.

A classic apoptotic cell death looks very different. In apoptosis, chromatin condenses and marginates to the nuclear membrane. Cell volume is reduced with notable crowding of morphological normal organelles, and membranes bleb to form apoptotic bodies [139–141]. In addition, all events occur in the absence of lymphocyte infiltration or exudative inflammation. Notable in the original descriptions of apoptosis was the specific citation of ischemia as a mechanism to produce coagulative necrosis.

The original descriptions of apoptosis occurred before the appreciation that there is a biology of cell death, complete with genetic, molecular, biochemical and macromolecular components. This raised the question of whether a biochemical apoptosis or programmed death could occur in the absence of apoptotic morphology. To this end, Schwartz et al. [142] compared the programmed cell death of the interstitial muscles in the moth, *Manduca sexta*, with the classical apoptotic death of thymocytes exposed to glucocorticoids. These two well-described models of active cell death displayed differences in cell surface morphology, nuclear ultrastructure and DNA fragmentation, suggesting the existence of tissue-specific morphology in physiologically programmed cell deaths.

Apoptotic Morphology in Stroke

The morphology of neurons during ischemia-induced death has been evaluated in global and focal models. A detailed study using light and electron microscopy was conducted to look for evidence of apoptosis in CA1 hippocampal neurons after 10 min of global ischemia [78]. These investigators reported that the most prominent early feature of delayed neuronal death was polysome disaggregation, and that the mitochondrial and nuclear elements remained intact until frank neuronal degeneration. The authors concluded that delayed neuronal death does not exhibit the prominent features of apoptosis.

In contrast, Nitatori et al. [143] recently examined delayed neuronal death in the CA1 pyramidal cell layer using similar approaches. These investigators reported that the mitochondria are intact when nuclear changes initiate and concluded that this cell death exhibits apoptotic morphology. Thus, the issue of whether apoptotic morphology occurs in global ischemia remains controversial and seems to largely revolve around the issue of whether chromatin condensation is a prominent feature of delayed neuronal death in CA1 hippocampal neurons.

The focal ischemia models produce a more rapid death that involves a large contiguous tract of cells and likely contains a core of frank necrotic cell death. Using light and electron microscopy methods, Li et al. [15, 23, 24, 144] have provided unambiguous data from isolated neurons that exhibited several classic features of apoptosis including chromatin aggregation, cytoplasmic condensation, and the appearance of apoptotic bodies containing fragments of condensed nuclear chromatin. These neurons tend to be found along the inner boundary zone of the infarction, suggesting that apoptosis is associated with those tissues that are amenable to pharmacological manipulation.

Future Directions

The term necrosis now appears inadequate to fully explain the cell death associated with stroke. However, the desire to classify ischemic cell death under the category of apoptosis is less important than recognizing that there is a biology of cell death that is activated by ischemia. Furthermore, it is important to recognize that ischemic cells respond to extracellular insults by intracellular mechanisms that include signal transduction, enzyme activation, and transcriptional regulation, and these responses are integral to determining the survival of a cell after a stroke.

An advanced understanding of cell death biology offers significant therapeutic opportunities. For example, the combined data suggests that ischemia initiates a cascade of intracellular events that eventually lead to an irreversible commitment to cell death. Inhibiting death at or before this commitment point may allow one to identify compounds that have an extended therapeutic window of opportunity relative to therapies that target earlier events in the ischemic sequelae. An extended window of opportunity would make it possible to provide therapeutic benefit to a greater percentage of the acute stroke patients.

Furthermore, if therapeutic approaches could be developed that prevent the commitment to cell death, ischemic cells may be persuaded to persist in a state of suspended animation until adequate reperfusion is provided. This type of therapy would offer the possibility of actually expanding the window of opportunity beyond normal physiological limits. While suspended animation has the potential to temporarily disrupt neuronal function, reperfusion may allow these neurons to recover function over time.

As in any new field, there are more questions than answers. However, apoptosis and cell death biology offer several new and compelling observations that help explain the pathophysiology associated with stroke and suggest novel therapeutic approaches for treating this disorder.

References

1 Oppenheim RW: Cell death during development of the nervous system. Annu Rev Neurosci 1991; 14:453–501.

2 Johnson EM Jr, Deckwerth TL: Molecular mechanisms of developmental neuronal death. Annu Rev Neurosci 1993;16:31–46.

3 Clark RK, Lee EV, White RF, Jonak ZL, Feuerstein GZ, Barone FC: Reperfusion following focal stroke hastens inflammation and resolution of ischemic injured tissue. Brain Res Bull 1994;35: 387–392.

4 Zhang RL, Chopp M, Chen H, Garcia JH: Temporal profile of ischemic tissue damage, neutrophil response, and vascular plugging following permanent and transient (2H) middle cerebral artery occlusion in the rat. J Neurol Sci 1994;125:3–10.

5 Barone FC, Schmidt DB, Hillegass LM, Price WJ, White RF, Feuerstein GZ, Clark RK, Lee EV, Griswold DE, Sarau HM: Reperfusion increases neutrophils and leukotriene B_4 receptor binding in rat focal ishcemia. Stroke 1992;23:1337–1347.

6 Garcia JH, Liu KF, Yoshida Y, Lian J, Chen S, del Zoppo GJ: Influx of leukocytes and platelets in an evolving brain infarct. Am J Pathol 1994;144:188–199.

7 Feuerstein GZ, Wang X, Barone FC: Inflammatory mediators and brain injury: The role of cytokines and chemokines in stroke and CNS disease; in Ginsberg MD, Bogousslavsky J (eds): Cerebrovascular Diseases. Cambridge, Blackwell Scientific, 1996.

8 Chopp M, Li Y, Zhang ZG, Freytag SO: p53 expression in brain after middle cerebral artery occlusion in the rat. Biochem Biophys Res Commun 1992;182:1201–1207.

9 Li Y, Chopp M, Zhang ZG, Zaloga C, Niewenhuis L, Gautam S: p53-immunoreactive protein and p53 mRNA expression after transient middle cerebral artery occlusion in rats. Stroke 1994;25: 849–856.

10 Martin SJ, Green DR: Protease activation during apoptosis: Death by a thousand cuts? Cell 1995; 82:349–352.

11 Xia Z, Dickens M, Raingeaud J, Davis RJ, Greenberg ME: Opposing effects of ERK and JNK-p38 MAP kinases on apoptosis. Science 1995;270:1326–1331.

12 Chopp M, Chan PH, Hsu CY, Cheung ME, Jacobs TP: DNA damage and repair in central nervous system injury. Stroke 1996;27:363–369.

13 Linnik MD, Zobrist RH, Hatfield MD: Evidence supporting a role for programmed cell death in focal cerebral ischemia in rats. Stroke 1993;24:2002–2009.

14 MacManus JP, Hill IE, Huang Z-G, Rasquinha I, Xue D, Buchan AM: DNA damage consistent with apoptosis in transient focal ischemic neocortex. Neuroreport 1994;5:493–496.
15 Li Y, Chopp M, Jiang N, Yao F, Zaloga C: Temporal profile of in situ DNA fragmentation after transient middle cerebral artery occlusion in the rat. J Cereb Blood Flow Metab 1995;15:389–397.
16 Linnik MD, Miller JA, Sprinkle-Cavallo J, Mason PJ, Thompson FY, Montgomery LR, Schroeder KK: Apoptotic DNA fragmentation in the rat cerebral cortex induced by permanent middle cerebral artery occlusion. Brain Res Mol Brain Res 1995;32:116–124.
17 Heron A, Pollard H, Dessi F, Moreau J, Lasbennes F, Ben-Ari Y, Charriaut-Marlangue C: Regional variability in DNA fragmentation after global ischemia evidenced by combined histological and gel electrophoresis observations in the rat brain. J Neurochem 1993;61:1973–1976.
18 MacManus JP, Buchan AM, Hill IE, Rasquinha I, Preston E: Global ischemia can cause DNA fragmentation indicative of apoptosis in rat brain. Neurosci Lett 1993;164:89–92.
19 Okamoto M, Matsumoto M, Ohtsuki T, Taguchi A, Mikoshiba K, Yanagihara T, Kamada T: Internucleosomal DNA cleavage involved in ischemia-induced neuronal death. Biochem Biophys Res Commun 1993;196:1356–1362.
20 Sei Y, Von Lubitz KJ, Basile AS, Borner MM, Lin RC, Skolnick P, Fossom LH: Internucleosomal DNA fragmentation in gerbil hippocampus following forebrain ischemia. Neurosci Lett 1994;171:179–182.
21 MacManus JP, Hill IE, Preston E, Rasquinha I, Walker T, Buchan AM: Differences in DNA fragmentation following transient cerebral or decapitation ischemia in rats. J Cereb Blood Flow Metab 1995;15:728–737.
22 Hill IE, MacManus JP, Rasquinha I, Tuor UI: DNA fragmentation indicative of apoptosis following unilateral cerebral hypoxia-ischemia in the neonatal rat. Brain Res 1995;676:398–403.
23 Li Y, Chopp M, Jiang N, Zhang ZG, Zaloga C: Induction of DNA fragmentation after 10 to 120 minutes of focal cerebral ischemia in rats. Stroke 1995;26:1252–1258.
24 Li Y, Chopp M, Jiang N, Zaloga C: In situ detection of DNA fragmentation after focal cerebral ischemia in mice. Brain Res Mol Brain Res 1995;28:164–168.
25 Charriaut-Marlangue C, Margaill I, Represa A, Popovici T, Plotkine M, Ben-Ari Y: Apoptosis and necrosis after reversible focal ischemia: An in situ DNA fragmentation analysis. J Cereb Blood Flow Metab 1996;16:186–194.
26 Gavrieli Y, Sherman Y, Ben-Sasson SA: Identification of programmed cell death in situ via specific labeling of nuclear DNA fragmentation. J Cell Biol 1992;119:493–501.
27 Walker PR, Sikorska M: Endonuclease activities, chromatin structure, and DNA degradation in apoptosis. Biochem Cell Biol 1994;72:615–623.
28 Walker PR, Weaver VM, Lach B, LeBlanc J, Sikorska M: Endonuclease activities associated with high molecular weight and internucleosomal DNA fragmentation in apoptosis. Exp Cell Res 1994;213:100–106.
29 Pandey S, Walker PR, Sikorska M: Separate pools of endonuclease activity are responsible for internucleosomal and high molecular mass DNA fragmentation during apoptosis. Biochem Cell Biol 1994;72:625–629.
30 Charriaut-Marlangue C, Margaill I, Plotkine M, Ben-Ari Y: Early endonuclease activation following reversible focal ischemia in the rat brain. J Cereb Blood Flow Metab 1995;15:385–388.
31 Fadok VA, Voelker DR, Campbell PA, Cohen JJ, Bratton DL, Henson PM: Exposure of phosphatidylserine on the surface of apoptotic lymphocytes triggers specific recognition and removal by macrophages. J Immunol 1992;148:2207–2216.
32 Sambrano GR, Steinberg D: Recognition of oxidatively damaged and apoptotic cells by an oxidized low density lipoprotein receptor on mouse peritoneal macrophages: Role of membrane phosphatidylserine. Proc Natl Acad Sci USA 1995;92:1396–1400.
33 Yuan Y, Shaham S, Ledoux S, Ellis HM, Horvitz HR: The *C. elegans* cell death gene ced-3 encodes a protein similar to mammalian interleukin-1β-converting enzyme. Cell 1993;75:641–652.
34 Thornberry NA: Interleukin-1-beta converting enzyme. Methods Enzymol 1994;244:615–631.
35 Gagliardini V, Fernandez P-A, Lee RKK, Drexler HCA, Rotello RJ, Fishman MC, Yuan J: Prevention of vertebrate neuronal death by the crmA gene. Science 1994;263:826–828.

36 Minami M, Kuraishi Y, Yabuuchi K, Yamazaki A, Satoh M: Induction of interleukin-1-beta mRNA in rat brain after transient forebrain ischemia. J Neurochem 1992;58:390–392.
37 Wang X, Yue TL, Barone FC, White RF, Gagnon RC, Feuerstein GZ: Concomitant cortical expression of TNF-alpha and IL-1-beta mRNAs follows early response gene expression in transient focal ischemia. Mol Chem Neuropathol 1994;23:103–114.
38 Yabuuchi K, Minami M, Katsumata S, Yamazaki A, Satoh M: An in situ hybridization study on interleukin-1-beta mRNA induced by transient forebrain ischemia in the rat brain. Brain Res Mol Brain Res 1994;26:135–142.
39 Buttini M, Sauter A, Boddeke HW: Induction of interleukin-1-beta mRNA after focal cerebral ischaemia in the rat. Brain Res Mol Brain Res 1994;23:126–134.
40 Betz AL, Yang GY, Davidson BL: Attenuation of stroke size in rats using an adenoviral vector to induce overexpression of interleukin-1 receptor antagonist in brain. J Cereb Blood Flow Metab 1995;15:547–551.
41 Yamasaki Y, Matsuura N, Shozuhara H, Onodera H, Itoyama Y, Kogure K: Interleukin-1 as a pathogenetic mediator of ischemic brain damage in rats. Stroke 1995;26:676–680.
42 Friedlander RM, Gagliardini V, Hara H, Moskowitz MA, Yuan J: Neuronal apoptosis following activation of the ICE family is mediated by secreted mature IL-1β. Am Assoc Neurol Surg Abstr, 1996, p 7.
43 Milligan CE, Prevette D, Yaginuma H, Homma S, Cardwell C, Fritz LC, Tomaselli KJ, Oppenheim RW, Schwartz LM: Peptide inhibitors of the ICE protease family arrest programmed cell death of motoneurons in vivo and in vitro. Neuron 1995;15:385–393.
44 Nicholson DW, Ali A, Thornberry NA, Vaillancourt JP, Ding CK, Gallant M, Gareau Y, Griffin PR, Labelle M, Lazebnik YA, Munday NA, Raju SM, Smulson ME, Yamin TT, Yu VL, Miller DK: Identification and inhibition of the ICE/CED-3 protease necessary for mammalian apoptosis. Nature 1995;376:37–43.
45 Kumar S: ICE-like proteases in apoptosis. Trends Biol Sci 1995;20:198–202.
46 Nicholson DW: ICE/CED3-like proteases as therapeutic targets for the control of inappropriate apoptosis. Nat Biotechnol 1996;14:297–301.
47 Wilson KP, Black JA, Thomson JA, Kim EE, Griffith JP, Navia MA, Murcko MA, Chambers SP, Aldape RA, Raybuck SA, Livingston DJ: Structure and mechanism of interleukin-1-beta converting enzyme. Nature 1994;370:270–275.
48 Sorimachi H, Tsukahara T, Okada-Ban M, Sugita H, Ishiura S, Suzuki K: Identification of a third ubiquitous calpain species – Chicken muscle expresses four distinct calpains. Biochim Biophys Acta 1995;1261:381–393.
49 Wang KKW, Yuen P-W: Calpain inhibition: An overview of its therapeutic potential. Trends Pharmacol Sci 1994;15:412–419.
50 Sorimachi H, Saido TC, Suzuki K: New era of calpain research. Discovery of tissue-specific calpains. FEBS Lett 1994;343:1–5.
51 Saido TC, Sorimachi H, Suzuki K: Calpain: New perspectives in molecular diversity and physiological-pathological involvement. FASEB J 1994;8:814–822.
52 Saito K, Elce JS, Hamos JE, Nixon RA: Widespread activation of calcium-activated neutral proteinase (calpain) in the brain in Alzheimer disease: A potential molecular basis for neuronal degeneration. Proc Natl Acad Sci USA 1993;90:2628–2632.
53 Kishimoto A, Mikawa K, Hashimoto K, Yasuda I, Tanaka S, Tominga M, Kuroda T, Nishizuka Y: Limited proteolysis of protein kinase C by calcium activated neutral proteinase (calpain). J Biol Chem 1989;264:4088–4092.
54 Squier MKT, Miller ACK, Malkinson AM, Cohen JJ: Calpain activation in apoptosis. J Cell Physiol 1994;159:229–237.
55 Sarin A, Adams DH, Henkart PA: Protease inhibitors selectively block T cell receptor-mediated programmed cell death in a murine T cell hybridoma and activated peripheral T cells. J Exp Med 1993;178:1693–1700.
56 Martin SJ, O'Brien GA, Nishioka WK, McGahon GA, Mahboubi A, Saido TC, Green DR: Proteolysis of fodrin (non-erythroid spectrin) during apoptosis. J Biol Chem 1995;270:6425–6428.

57 Martin DP, Ito A, Horigome K, Lampe PA, Johnson EM: Biochemical characterization of programmed cell death in NGF-deprived sympathetic neurons. J Neurobiol 1992;23:1205–1220.
58 Pittman RN, Wang S, DiBenedetto AJ, Mills JC: A system for characterizing cellular and molecular events in programmed neuronal cell death. J Neurosci 1993;13:3669–3680.
59 D'Mello SR, Galli C, Ciotti T, Calissano P: Induction of apoptosis in cerebellar granule neurons by low potassium: Inhibition of death by insulin growth factor I and cAMP. Proc Natl Acad Sci USA 1993;90:10989–10993.
60 Sarin A, Nakajima H, Henkart PA: A protease-dependent TCR-induced death pathway in mature lymphocytes. J Immunol 1995;154:5806–5812.
61 Siman R, Noszek JC: Excitatory amino acids activate calpain I and induce structural protein breakdown in vivo. Neuron 1988;1:279–287.
62 Siman R, Roszek JC, Kegerise C: Calpain I activation is specifically related to excitatory amino acid induction of hippocampal damage. J Neurosci 1989;9:1579–1590.
63 Bartus RT, Dean RL, Cavanaugh K, Eveleth D, Carriero DL, Lynch G: Time-related neuronal changes following middle cerebral artery occlusion: Implications for therapeutic intervention and the role of calpain. J Cereb Blood Flow Metab 1995;15:969–979.
64 Yao H, Ginsberg MD, Eveleth DD, LaManna JC, Watson BD, Alonso OF, Loor JY, Foreman JH, Busto R: Local cerebral glucose utilization and cytoskeletal proteolysis as indices of evolving focal ischemic injury in core and penumbra. J Cereb Blood Flow Metab 1995;15:398–408.
65 Hong S-C, Goto Y, Lanzino G, Soleau S, Kassell NF, Lee KS: Neuroprotection with a calpain inhibitor in a model of focal cerebral ischemia. Stroke 1994;25:663–669.
66 Lee KS, Frank S, Vanderklish P, Arai A, Lynch G: Inhibition of proteolysis protects hippocampal neurons from ischemia. Proc Natl Acad Sci USA 1991;88:7233–7237.
67 Yokota M, Saido TC, Tani E, Kawashima S, Suzuki K: Three distinct phases of fodrin proteolysis induced in postischemic hippocampus. Involvement of calpain and unidentified protease. Stroke 1995;26:1901–1907.
68 Rami A, Krieglstein J: Protective effects of calpain inhibitors against neuronal damage caused by cytotoxic hypoxia in vitro and ischemia in vivo. Brain Res 1993;609:67–70.
69 Arai A, Kessler M, Lee K, Lynch G: Calpain inhibitors improve the recovery of synaptic transmission from hypoxia in hippocampal slices. Brain Res 1990;532:63–68.
70 Bartus RT, Hayward NJ, Elliott PJ, Sawyer SD, Baker KL, Dean RL, Akiyama A, Straub JA, Harbeson SL, Li Z, Powers J: Calpain inhibitor AK295 protects neurons from focal brain ischemia. Stroke 1994;25:2265–2270.
71 Bartus RT, Baker KL, Heiser AD, Sawyer SD, Dean RL, Elliott PJ, Straub JA: Postischemic administration of AK275, a calpain inhibitor, provides substantial protection against focal ischemic brain damage. J Cereb Blood Flow Metab 1994;14:537–544.
72 Yoshizawa T, Sorimachi H, Tomioka S, Ishiura S, Suzuki K: A catalytic subunit of calpain possesses full proteolytic activity. FEBS Lett 1995;358:101–103.
73 Martin DP, Schmidt RE, DiStefano PS, Lowry OH, Carter JG, Johnson EM Jr: Inhibitors of protein synthesis and RNA synthesis prevent neuronal death caused by nerve growth factor deprivation. J Cell Biol 1988;106:829–844.
74 Goto K, Ishige A, Sekiguchi K, Iizuka S, Sugimoto A, Yuzurihara M, Aburada M, Hosoya E, Kogure K: Effects of cycloheximide on delayed neuronal death in rat hippocampus. Brain Res 1990; 534:299–302.
75 Shigeno T, Yamasaki Y, Kato G, Kausaka K, Mima T, Takakura K, Graham DI, Furukawa S: Reduction of delayed neuronal death by inhibition of protein synthesis. Neurosci Lett 1990;120: 117–119.
76 Papas S, Crepel V, Hasboun D, Jorquera I, Chinestra P, Ben-Ari Y: Cycloheximide reduces the effects of anoxic insult in vivo and in vitro. Eur J Neurosci 1992;4:758–765.
77 Kiessling M, Xie Y, Ullrich B, Thilmann R: Are the neuroprotective effects of the protein synthesis inhibitor cycloheximide due to the prevention of apoptosis? J Cereb Blood Flow Metab 1991;11:S357.
78 Deshpande J, Bergstedt K, Linden T, Kalimo H, Wieloch T: Ultrastructural changes in the hippocampal CA1 region following transient cerebral ischemia: Evidence against programmed cell death. Exp Brain Res 1992;88:91–105.

79 Du C, Hu R, Csernansky CA, Hsu CY, Choi DW: Very delayed infarction after mild focal cerebral ischemia: A role for apoptosis? J Cereb Blood Flow Metab 1996;16:195–201.

80 Estus S, Zaks WJ, Freeman RS, Gruda M, Bravo R, Johnson EM: Altered gene expression in neurons during programmed cell death: Identification of c-jun as necessary for neuronal apoptosis. J Cell Biol 1994;127:1717–1727.

81 Hsu CY, An G, Liu JS, Xue JJ, He YY, Lin TN: Expression of immediate early gene and growth factor mRNAs in a focal cerebral ischemia model in the rat. Stroke 1993;24:I78–I81.

82 Wang X, Yue T-L, Young PR, Barone FC, Feuerstein GZ: Expression of interleukin-6, c-fos, and zif268 mRNAs in rat ischemic cortex. J Cereb Blood Flow Metab 1995;15:166–171.

83 Onodera H, Kogure K, Ono Y, Igarashi K, Kiyota Y, Nagaoka A: Proto-onocogene c-fos is transiently induced in the rat cerebral cortex after forebrain ischemia. Neurosci Lett 1989;98:101–104.

84 Collaco-Moraes Y, Aspey BS, de Belleroche JS, Harrison MJG: Focal ischemia causes an extensive induction of immediate early genes that are sensitive to MK-801. Stroke 1994;25:1855–1861.

85 Neumann-Haefelin T, Wiessner C, Vogel P, Back T, Hossmann KA: Differential expression of the immediate early genes c-fos, c-jun, junB, and NGFI-B in the rat brain following transient forebrain ischemia. J Cereb Blood Flow Metab 1994;14:206–216.

86 Kinouchi H, Sharp FR, Chan PH, Koistinaho J, Sagar SM, Yoshimoto T: Induction of c-fos, junB, c-jun, and hsp70 mRNA in cortex, thalamus, basal ganglia, and hippocampus following middle cerebral artery occlusion. J Cereb Blood Flow Metab 1994;14:808–817.

87 Honkaniemi J, Sagar SM, Pyykonen I, Hicks KJ, Sharp FR: Focal brain injury induces multiple immediate early genes encoding zinc finger transcription factors. Brain Res Mol Brain Res 1995; 28:157–163.

88 Freeman RS, Estus S, Johnson EM: Analysis of cell cycle-related gene expression in postmitotic neurons: Selective induction of cyclin D1 during programmed cell death. Neuron 1994;12:343–355.

89 Liu PK, Salminen A, He YY, Jiang MH, Xue JJ, Liu JS, Hsu CY: Suppression of ischemia-induced fos expression and AP-1 activity by an antisense oligodeoxynucleotide to c-fos mRNA. Ann Neurol 1994;36:566–576.

90 Martinou JC, Dubois-Dauphin M, Staple JK, Rodriguez I, Frankowski H, Missotten M, Albertini P, Talabot D, Catsicas S, Pietra C, Huarte J: Overexpression of BCL-2 in transgenic mice protects neurons from naturally occurring cell death and experimental ischemia. Neuron 1994;13:1017–1030.

91 Crumrine RC, Thomas AL, Morgan PF: Attenuation of p53 expression protects against focal ischemic damage in transgenic mice. J Cereb Blood Flow Metab 1994;14:887–891.

92 Yang G, Chan PH, Chen J, Carlson E, Chen SF, Weinstein P, Epstein CJ, Kamii H: Human copper-zinc superoxide dismutase transgenic mice are highly resistant to reperfusion injury after focal cerebral ischemia. Stroke 1994;25:165–170.

93 Huang PL, Huang Z, Mashimo H, Bloch KD, Moskowitz MA, Bevan JA, Fishman MC: Hypertension in mice lacking the gene for endothelial nitric oxide synthase. Nature 1995;377:239–242.

94 Linnik MD, Zahos P, Geschwind MD, Federoff HJ: Expression of bcl-2 from a defective herpes simplex virus 1 vector limits neuronal death in focal cerebral ischemia. Stroke 1995;26:1670–1675.

95 Lawrence MS, Ho DY, Sun GH, Steinberg GK, Sapolsky RM: Overexpression of Bcl-2 with herpes simplex virus vectors protects CNS neurons against neurological insults in vitro and in vivo. J Neurosci 1996;16:486–496.

96 Lawrence MS, Sun GH, Kunis DM, Saydam TC, Dash R, Ho DY, Sapolsky RM, Steinberg GK: Overexpression of the glucose transporter gene with a herpes simplex viral vector protects striatal neurons against stroke. J Cereb Blood Flow Metab 1996;16:181–185.

97 Tsujimoto Y, Finger LR, Yunis J, Nowell PC, Croce CM: Cloning of the chromosome brakepoint of neoplastic B cells with the t(14;18) chromosome translocation. Science 1984;226:1097–1099.

98 Tsujimoto Y, Croce CM: Analysis of the structure, transcripts, and protein products of bcl-2, the gene involved in human follicular lymphoma. Proc Natl Acad Sci USA 1986;83:5214–5218.

99 Hengartner MO, Ellis RE, Horvitz HR: *Caenorhabditis elegans* gene ced-9 protects cells from programmed cell death. Nature 1992;356:494–499.

100 Vaux DL, Weissman IL, Kim SK: Prevention of programmed cell death in *Caenorhabditis elegans* by human bcl-2. Science 1992;258:1955–1957.

101 Hengartner MO, Horvitz HR: *C. elegans* cell survival gene ced-9 encodes a functional homolog of the mammalian proto-oncogene bcl-2. Cell 1994;76:665–676.
102 Reed JC; Bcl-2 and the regulation of programmed cell death. J Cell Biol 1994;124:1–6.
103 Bredesen DE: Neural Apoptosis. Ann Neurol 1995;38:839–851.
104 Kane DJ, Ord T, Anton R, Bredesen DE: Expression of bcl-2 inhibits necrotic neural cell death. J Neurosci Res 1995;40:269–275.
105 Behl C, Hovey L III, Krajewski S, Schubert D, Reed JC: Bcl-2 prevents killing of neuronal cells by glutamate but not by amyloid beta protein. Biochem Biophys Res Commun 1993;197:949–956.
106 Zhong LT, Kane DJ, Bredesen DE: Bcl-2 blocks glutamate toxicity in neural cell lines. Brain Res Mol Brain Res 1993;19:353–355.
107 Zhong L-T, Sarafian T, Kane DJ, Charles AC, Mah SP, Edwards RH, Bredesen DE: bcl-2 inhibits death of central neural cells induced by multiple agents. Proc Natl Acad Sci USA 1993;90:4533–4537.
108 Hockenbery DM, Oltvai ZN, Yin X-M, Milliman CL, Korsmeyer SJ: Bcl-2 functions in an antioxidant pathway to prevent apoptosis. Cell 1993;75:241–251.
109 Kane DJ, Sarafian TA, Anton R, Hahn H, Gralla EB, Valentine JS, Örd T, Bredesen DE: Bcl-2 inhibition of neural death: Decreased generation of reactive oxygen species. Science 1993;262:1274–1277.
110 Jacobson MD, Raff MC: Programmed cell death and bcl-2 protection in very low oxygen. Nature 1995;374:814–816.
111 Shimizu S, Eguchi Y, Kosaka H, Kamiike W, Matsuda H, Tsujimoto Y: Prevention of hypoxia-induced cell death by Bcl-2 and Bcl-xL. Nature 1995;374:811–813.
112 Myers KM, Fiskum G, Liu Y, Simmens SJ, Bredesen DE, Murphy AN: Bcl-2 protects neural cells from cyanide/aglycemia-induced lipid oxidation, mitochondrial injury, and loss of viability. J Neurochem 1995;65:2432–2440.
113 Merry DE, Veis DJ, Hickey WF, Korsmeyer SJ: bcl-2 protein expression is widespread in the developing nervous system and retained in the adult PNS. Development 1994;120:301–311.
114 Castren E, Ohga Y, Berzaghi MP, Tzimagiorgis G, Thoenen H, Lindholm D: bcl-2 messenger RNA is localized in neurons of the devoloping and adult rat brain. Neuroscience 1994;61:165–177.
115 Krajewski S, Mai JK, Sikorska M, Mossakowski MJ, Reed JC: Upregulation of Bax protein levels in neurons following cerebral ischemia. J Neurosci 1995;15:6364–6376.
116 Chen J, Graham SH, Chan PH, Lan J, Zhou RL, Simon RP: bcl-2 is expressed in neurons that survive focal ischemia in the rat. Neuroreport 1995;6:394–398.
117 Shimazaki K, Ishida A, Kawai N: Increase in bcl-2 oncoprotein and the tolerance to ischemia-induced neuronal death in the gerbil hippocampus. Neurosci Res 1994;20:95–99.
118 Nunez G, Clarke MF: The bcl-2 family of proteins: Regulators of cell death and survival. Trends Cell Biol 1994;4:399–403.
119 Davies AM: The bcl-2 family of proteins, and the regulation of neuronal survival. Trends Neurol Sci 1995;18:355–358.
120 Yin XM, Oltval ZN, Kormeyer SJ: BH1 and BH2 domains of Bcl-2 are required for inhibition of apoptosis and heterodimerization with Bax. Nature 1994;369:272–273.
121 Sedlak TW, Oltvai ZN, Yang E, Wang K, Boise LH, Thompson CB, Korsmeyer SJ: Multiple Bcl-2 family members demonstrate selective dimerizations with Bax. Proc Natl Acad Sci USA 1995;92:7834–7838.
122 Yang E, Zha J, Jockel J, Boise LH, Thompson CB, Korsmeyer SJ: Bad, a heterodimeric partner for Bcl-XL and Bcl-2, displaces Bax and promotes cell death. Cell 1995;80:285–291.
123 Boise LH, Gonzalez-Garcia M, Postema CE, Ding L, Lindsten T, Turka LA, Mao X, Nunez G, Thompson CB: bcl-x, a bcl-2-related gene that functions as a dominant regulator of apoptotic cell death. Cell 1993;74:597–608.
124 Gonzalez-Garcia M, Garcia I, Ding L, O'Shea S, Boise LH, Thompson CB, Nunez G: bcl-x is expressed in embryonic and postnatal neural tissues and functions to prevent neuronal cell death. Proc Natl Acad Sci USA 1995;92:4304–4308.
125 Oltvai ZN, Milliman CL, Korsmeyer SJ: Bcl-2 heterodimerizes in vivo with a conserved homolog, bax, that accelerates programmed cell death. Cell 1993;74:609–619.

126 Hockenbery DM, Nunez G, Milliman C, Schreiber RD, Korsmeyer SJ: Bcl-2 is an inner mitochondrial membrane protein that blocks programmed cell death. Nature 1990;348:334–336.
127 Alnemri ES, Robertson NM, Fernandes TF, Croce CM, Litwack G: Overexpressed full-length human Bcl-2 extends survival of baculovirus-infected SF9 insect cells. Proc Natl Acad Sci USA 1992;89:7295–7299.
128 Newmeyer DD, Farschon DM, Reed JC: Cell-free apoptosis in Xenopus egg extracts: Inhibition by Bcl-2 and requirement for an organelle fraction enriched in mitochondria. Cell 1994;79:353–364.
129 Jacobson MD, Burne JF, King MP, Miyashita T, Reed JC, Raff MC: Bcl-2 blocks apoptosis in cells lacking mitochondrial DNA. Nature 1993;361:365–369.
130 Cheng EHY, Levine B, Boise LH, Thompson CB, Hardwick JM: Bax-independent inhibition of apoptosis by bcl-xl. Nature 1996;379:554–556.
131 Yonish-Rouach E, Grunwald D, Wilder S, Kimchi A, May E, Lawrence JJ, May P, Oren M: p53-mediated cell death: Relationship to cell cycle control. Mol Cell Biol 1993;13:1415–1423.
132 Lowe SW, Ruley HE, Jacks T, Housman DE: p53-dependent apoptosis modulates the cytotoxicity of anticancer agents. Cell 1993;74:957–967.
133 Symonds H, Krall L, Remington L, Saenz-Robles M, Lowe S, Jacks T, Van Dyke T: p53-dependent apoptosis suppresses tumor growth and progression in vivo. Cell 1994;78:703–711.
134 Sakhi A, Bruce A, Sun N, Tocco G, Baudry M, Schreiber SS: p53 induction is associated with neuronal damage in the central nervous system. Proc Natl Acad Sci USA 1994;91:7525–7529.
135 Wood KA, Youle RJ: The role of free radicals and p53 in neuron apoptosis in vivo. J Neurosci 1995;15:5851–5857.
136 Morrison RS, Wenzel HJ, Kinoshita Y, Robbins CA, Donehower LA, Schwartzkroin PA: Loss of the p53 tumor suppressor gene protects neurons from kainate-induced cell death. J Neurosci 1996;16:1337–1345.
137 Wang Y, Okan I, Szekely L, Klein G, Wiman KG: bcl-2 inhibits wild-type p53-triggered apoptosis but not G1 cell cycle arrest and transactivation of WAF1 and bax. Cell Growth Differ 1995;6:1071–1075.
138 Schott AF, Apel IJ, Nunez G, Clarke MF: Bcl-XL protects cancer cells from p53-mediated apoptosis. Oncogene 1995;11:1389–1394.
139 Kerr JFR, Wyllie AH, Currie AR: Apoptosis: A basic biological phenomenon with wide ranging implications in tissue kinetics. Br J Cancer 1972;26:239–257.
140 Wyllie AH, Kerr JFR, Currie AR: Cell death: The significance of apoptosis. Int Rev Cytol 1980;68:251–306.
141 Kerr JFR, Gobe GC, Winterford CM, Harmon BV: Anatomical methods in cell death. Methods Cell Biol 1995;46:1–27.
142 Schwartz LM, Smith SW, Jones MEE, Osborne BA: Do all programmed cell deaths occur via apoptosis? Proc Natl Acad Sci USA 1993;90:980–984.
143 Nitatori T, Sato N, Waguri S, Karasawa Y, Araki H, Shibanai K, Kominami E, Uchiyama Y: Delayed neuronal death in the CA1 pyramidal cell layer of the gerbil hippocampus following transient ischemia is apoptosis. J Neurosci 1995;15:1001–1011.
144 Li Y, Sharov VG, Jiang N, Zaloga C, Sabbah HN, Chopp M: Ultrastructural and light microscopic evidence of apoptosis after middle cerebral artery occlusion in the rat. Am J Pathol 1995;146:1045–1051.

Matthew D. Linnik, PhD, Hoechst Marion Roussel, Inc.,
2110 East Galbraith Road, Cincinnati, OH 45215-6300 (USA)

Hsu CY (ed): Ischemic Stroke: From Basic Mechanisms to New Drug Development.
Monogr Clin Neurosci. Basel, Karger, 1998, vol 16, pp 116–126

Neurotrophic Factors

Ke Chen, Seth P. Finklestein

CNS Growth Factor Research Laboratory, Department of Neurology,
Massachusetts General Hospital, and Harvard Medical School, Boston, Mass., USA

Neurotrophic growth factors are naturally-occurring polypeptides that, acting through high-affinity receptors, promote neuronal survival, and, in some cases, neuronal outgrowth as well. As a corollary, neurotrophic factors can protect neurons against a number of exogenous toxins and insults [1–3]. Several identified growth factors have neurotrophic and neuroprotective activities, including members of the fibroblast growth factor (FGF), neurotrophin, transforming growth factor-β (TGF-β), and insulin-like growth factor (IGF) superfamilies. The expression of many of these growth factors is up-regulated during brain development and after brain injury or stroke [4].

The molecular mechanisms of growth factor neurotrophism and neuroprotection are incompletely understood. It appears that, through interaction with high-affinity (generall tyrosine kinase) receptors, growth factors initiate cascades of signal transduction resulting in the expression of survival-promoting and protective genes and their products ('programmed cell life') [3]. Such gene products may include free radical scavenging enzymes, calcium binding proteins, and 'anti-apoptotic' proteins [3, 5].

Abundant evidence suggests that some brain neurons undergo a 'delayed' death following cerebral ischemia. These include 'selectively vulnerable' neurons following *global* ischemia, as well as neurons at the margins ('penumbra') of infarcts following *focal* ischemia [6, 7]. Mechanisms of delayed cell death after ischemia may include excitatory amino acid toxicity, free radical-induced damage, nitric oxide (NO) toxicity, and 'programmed' cell death (apoptosis) [8]. The occurrence of delayed cell death offers the opportunity of pharmacological therapy to 'rescue' vulnerable cells following ischemia. Because of their trophic/protective properties, growth factors have been considered as a possible pharmacological strategy to limit cell death after stroke. Moreover, because of their properties in enhancing neuronal outgrowth and synapse formation, growth factors have also been investigated as agents that might enhance functional recovery after ischemic cerebral damage has occurred.

Within the past few years, the availability of recombinant proteins has made possible the study of the effects of exogenously-administered growth factors in experimental models of stroke. The following chapter will summarize recent preclinical work on growth factor treatment of stroke, with emphasis on the FGF, neurotrophin, TGF-β, and IGF families. In comparing these studies, especially from the point of view of potential clinical applicability, it is important to take note of the age and species of animals; the specific ischemia models used; the dose, route, and timing of growth factor administration, and effects on the acute or recovery phases of stroke. In particular, some studies have been done using models of *global* cerebral ischemia, produced by temporary bilateral occlusion of cerebral arteries (ususally the carotids ± vertebrals) and resulting in the delayed death of selectively vulnerable brain neurons (e.g., in CA-1 hippocampus). Global ischemia models parallel the clinical condition of cardiac arrest. On the other hand, in models of *focal* cerebral ischemia, a unilateral arterial occlusion is made (generally of the middle cerebral artery (MCA)), resulting in a region of focal necrosis of all cells (infarct) within the territory supplied by the occluded artery. The arterial occlusion may be *permanent* (non-reperfusion) or temporary, resulting in *ischemia/reperfusion*. Alternatively, a focal infarct may be made by occlusion of a large extracranial artery (e.g., the carotid), combined with temporary exposure of the animal to a low oxygen environment (combined *hypoxia/ischemia* model). Models of focal ischemia parallel the common clinical condition of thromboembolic stroke. Because growth factors are proteins that do not normally cross the blood-brain barrier (BBB), these factors have generally been given intracerebroventricularly or intracisternally in preclinical studies of cerebral ischemia. However, because of evidence suggesting that systemically-administered growth factors may cross the damaged BBB after ischemia, recent studies have also utilized intraperitoneal or intravenous administration of factors.

Fibroblast Growth Factors

FGFs comprise a family of seven structurally-related proteins [9]. Of particular importance to the nervous system are acidic and basic FGF [10]. Acidic FGF (aFGF, FGF-1) is a 16-kD polypeptide and basic FGF (bFGF, FGF-2) is an 18-kD polypeptide that are found in the mature mammalian brain and are up-regulated during brain development and following injury or stroke [4, 11, 12]. These factors bind to a family of four high-affinity tyrosine kinase receptors (FGFR1–4). The FGFs have multipotential trophic effects on brain cells. Both aFGF and bFGF support the survival of brain neurons, glia, and endothelial cells, and are mitogens for glia and endothelia [10].

Basic FGF is the most extensively studied polypeptide growth factor in preclinical studies of stroke. This factor has potent survival-promoting effects on neurons from a number of regions of embryonic rat brain [13]. Moreover, bFGF protects cultured neurons against a number of exogenous toxins and insults, including anoxia, hypoglycemia, excitatory amino acids, free radicals, and NO [14–19]. The mechanism of bFGF-induced neuroprotection has not been fully elucidated, but appears to depend on new gene transcription and protein synthesis [14]. In neuronal culture, bFGF up-regulates the expression of free radical scavenging enzymes and calcium binding proteins, and down-regulates the expression of an NMDA receptor protein [2, 20]. In vivo in rat brain, bFGF is also a potent cerebral vasodilator, an effect that is mediated through NO-dependent mechanisms [21, 22].

Because of its cytoprotective as well as its vasoactive properties in brain, bFGF is a particularly promising agent to study in experimental models of stroke. In early studies [23, 24], the protective effects of bFGF were assessed in models of acute excitotoxicity in neonatal rats. Excitotoxic lesions were made in P7 rat pups by direct intrastriatal injections of NMDA. Animals received intraperitoneal injections of bFGF (50–300 μg/kg) or vehicle 30 min before lesions were made. Intraperitoneal bFGF treatment was associated with a dose-dependent decrease in the volume of excitotoxic lesions. Maximal reduction (ca. 40%) was achieved at a dose of 100 μg/kg. This reduction was augmented (to 60%) by multiple (three) bFGF injections given both before and after lesions were made. Significant reduction in lesion volume was also seen when a single intraperitoneal bFGF injection was made up to 1 h after excitotoxic lesions were made. This therapeutic time window is equivalent to that achieved by NMDA receptor antagonists in this model. Studies using labeled bFGF show that, in neonatal rats, intraperitoneally administered bFGF crosses the damaged BBB to enter the lesioned but not the intact cerebral hemisphere [25].

In companion studies [23], the protective effects of bFGF was tested in a model of focal hypoxic/ischemic infarction in neonatal rat brain. Pretreatment with intraperitoneal bFGF (100 μg/kg) reduced infarct volume by 40%; this effect was enhanced to 60% by multiple bFGF injections, both before and after the onset of ischemia.

'Proof of principle' of the protective effects of bFGF in a model of focal ischemia in mature rats was obtained in studies in which bFGF (1 μg/day) was administered by continuous intraventricular infusion for 3 days before focal infarcts were made by permanent unilateral middle cerebral artery occlusion (MCAO) and temporary bilateral common carotid artery occlusion (CCAO) [26]. At 24 h after ischemia, infarcts were smaller (by 25%) in bFGF-compared to vehicle-treated animals. In more recent studies of focal ischemia in mature rats, bFGF was delivered intravenously at times following the onset of focal ischemia. In a model of permanent MCAO by intraluminal suture occlusion, bFGF was administered by continuous intravenous infusion (45 μg/kg/h) at 0.5–3.5 h after ischemia [27]. In a model of focal ischemia/reperfusion, bFGF was delivered at this same dose for 3 h, starting at the time of reperfusion at 2 h after the onset of ischemia [28]. In both of these studies, a 40–50% reduction in infarct volume was found in bFGF-treated animals. These animals also had a corresponding reduction in the degree of sensorimotor disability after ischemia. Studies using a permanent MCAO model show that intravenously administered labeled bFGF crosses the damaged BBB to enter the ischemic, but not the nonischemic hemisphere [27]. Following permanent MCAO in rats, the effective bFGF dose is 5.0–50 μg/kg/h for 3 h, and the effective time window for initiation of treatment lasts up to 3 h after the onset of ischemia [29, Ren and Finklestein, unpubl. data].

In a rat model of permanent MCAO, reduction in infarct volume has also been reported following administration of bFGF (100 ng) by intracarotid bolus [30]. The infarct-reducing effects of bFGF have also been demonstrated in a model of focal ischemia in cats. Following permanent MCAO, intravenous infusion of bFGF at 5.0 μg/kg/h for 3 h reduced infarct volume by 50%; no further reduction in infarct size was obtained at doses of 50 or 250 μg/kg/h [31].

The mechanism of infarct reduction by systemically-adminstered bFGF following focal ischemia requires further study. In particular, the relative contribution of changes in regional cerebral blood flow (rCBF) versus direct cytoprotection requires clarification. In rats, studies using laser Doppler flowmetry show that intravenously or intra-arterially administered bFGF increases rCBF in the 'ischemic penumbra' surrounding focal infarcts [29, 30]. On the other hand, in cats, studies using microsphere methods show no increases in rCBF in the ischemic penumbra following bFGF administration [31]. Nonetheless, studies in both species show robust reductions in infarct size following intravenous bFGF [27, 28, 31]. This apparent paradox has been addressed in recent studies using genetically altered 'knockout' mice lacking the endothelial form of nitric oxide synthase (eNOS). As noted above, the vasodilatory effects of bFGF in rodents are mediated via NO [21, 32]. Thus, unlike wild-type mice, eNOS-deficient mice undergoing MCAO show no increase in rCBF in the ischemic penumbra following intravenous bFGF infusion [33]. On the other hand, the degree of infarct reduction is equivalent in eNOS-deficient and wild-type animals. These data, as well as the data obtained in cats [31], suggest that the mechanism of infarct reduction by intravenous bFGF is independent of changes in rCBF. An alternative mechanism is direct cytoprotection. As noted above, systemically-adminstered bFGF crosses the damaged BBB following injury or ischemia [25, 27] where it may become directly available to cell-associated high-affinity receptors, triggering signal transduction cascades resulting in cytoprotective gene expression. Clearly, since focal infarcts involve all cell types (including neurons, glia, and vascular cells), bFGF must protect all of these cells, either directly, through stimulation of its own receptors, or indirectly, through stimulation of other trophic factors. The expression of putative protective gene products following intravenous bFGF administration in models of focal ischemia is currently under active study.

In addition to the effects of bFGF in reducing infarct size following acute cerebral ischemia, recent studies show that this factor also promotes neurological recovery when delivered at longer times after ischemia. Mechanisms of functional recovery after focal brain injury or infarction are likely to include new axonal and dendritic sprouting and new synapse formation in the intact undamaged brain [34, 35]. As noted above, bFGF promotes both the survival and outgrowth of brain neurons in vitro [13]. Because of these properties, the effects of bFGF in promoting functional recovery has been tested in an animal model of focal cerebral infarction. bFGF (1 μg) or vehicle were administered by intracisternal injection twice weekly for 4 weeks following permanent unilateral MCAO in mature rats [36]. Animals were assessed using standard behavioral tests to determine forelimb, hindlimb, vestibular, and extrapyramidal function. At 1 month after infarction, animals were sacrificed. Infarct volume in the ipsilateral cortex and underlying striatum was not different between bFGF- and vehicle-treated animals, consistent with delivery of bFGF beyond the 'therapeutic window' for infarct reduction. There was, however, a marked enhancement of behavioral recovery in bFGF-treated animals that was particularly evident for tests of sensorimotor function of the affected (contralateral) forelimb and hindlimb. Intracisternal injection was chosen as the route of administration in these studies so that bFGF might gain access to the intact contralateral cortex, which may mediate functional recovery [35]. At the dose given (1 μg/injection; 8 μg total) intracisternal bFGF administration was associated with weight loss. In subsequent studies at lower doses, effects on behavioral recovery were preserved, without changes in body weight [Kawamata and Finklestein, unpubl. observations].

The mechanisms of enhanced behavioral recovery by intracisternal bFGF include protection against 'retrograde' neuronal death, as well as stimulation of new neuronal outgrowth and synapse formation. Intracisternal injection of bFGF (1 μg/week × 4 weeks) beginning at 1 day following focal infarction protects against the 'retrograde' death of thalamic neurons projecting to infarcted cortex [37]. Distant neurons surviving retrograde death in thalamus and elsewhere may ultimately make new synaptic connections contributing to functional recovery. In addition, intracisternal bFGF may promote local sprouting from neurons in cortex contralateral to infarcts, which may also contribute to functional recovery [35].

Although fewer studies have been done using a FGF in models of cerebral ischemia, at least two studies have shown that intraventricular aFGF protects against CA-1 neuronal death in models of global ischemia [38, 39]. In models of focal ischemia, intraventricular administration of aFGF spares cholinergic neurons projecting to infarcted cortex [40].

Neurotrophins

The neurotrophins comprise a family of at least four structurally related peptides, including NGF, BDNF, NT-3, and NT-4/5 [1, 41]. The neurotrophins bind to a low-affinity receptor (p75) as well as to a family of high-affinity tyrosine kinase receptors (the *trk* family). The prototypical neurotrophin, NGF, is a 26-kD homodimer that binds to the *trkA* receptor and has trophic effects on cholinergic neurons in the intact mature brain. BDNF is a 13-kD monomer that binds to the *trkB* receptor and has a wider spectrum of activity in the intact brain, including on cerebellar, hippocampal, cholinergic, and dopaminergic neurons.

NGF is the most extensively studied neurotrophin in models of neuroprotection. In vitro, NGF protects PC-12 cells against death from anoxia, and protects PC-12 cells as well as embryonic neurons from rat hippocampus and human cortex against hypoglycemia- and free radical-induced death [17, 19, 42, 43]. In in vivo models of global forebrain ischemia in gerbils and rats, the intraventricular administration of NGF (2–10 μg) beginning just before or just after the onset of ischemia has been reported to reduce death of CA-1 hippocampal neurons [44, 45], although this result has not been obtained by all investigators [46]. Other studies show that systemic treatment with *L*-threo-3,4-dihydroxyphenylserine (DOPS) and bezaseride, a strategy designed to increase NGF levels in brain, also reduces CA-1 neuronal loss following global forebrain ischemia in gerbils [47]. Moreover, local implantation of genetically altered fibroblasts secreting NGF also reduces neuronal death in hippocampus following global ischemia [48].

Fewer studies have been done regarding NGF treatment in models of focal ischemia. In neonatal rats, the intraventricular administration of NGF (15 μg) both before and after ischemia reduces infarct volume in a model of focal hypoxia/ischemia [49]. The intraventricular or local administration of

NGF also protects against the 'retrograde' death of distant cholinergic neurons in nucleus basalis projecting to infarcted cortex [50, 51].

It is not clear how NGF protects hippocampal or cortical neurons in following global or focal ischemia, since these neurons do not normally express low-affinity (p75) or high-affinity (*trkA*) receptors in the intact mature brain. On the other hand, there is evidence that brain injury or ischemia may upregulate the expression of NGF receptors (especially the p75 receptor) on neurons that do not normally express these receptors [47].

In addition to the above studies on NGF, at least one study shows that intraventricular BDNF reduces neuronal loss following global forebrain ischemia in gerbils [52].

Transforming Growth Factor-βs

The TGF-β superfamily includes TGF-βs 1–3, as well as activin/inhibin, the bone morphogenic proteins (BMPs), and several other identified growth factors [41, 53]. The prototypical TGF-β, TGF-β_1, is a homodimer of two 12-kD polypeptides. TGF-β_1 protects embryonic rat cerebrocortical neurons against glutamate toxicity and protects embryonic chick telencephalic neurons against glutamate toxicity and cytotoxic hypoxia in vitro [54, 55].

In models of permanent focal ischemia in mice or rabbits, pretreatment with intraventricular or intra-arterial TGF-β_1 reduced infarct volume [54, 56]. However, in a rabbit model, posttreatment with intra-arterial TGF-β_1 at 30 min after the onset of ischemia failed to reduce infarct size [57]. Intraventricular TGF-β_1 has been reported to reduce infarct volume when administered at 2 h following focal hypoxia/ischemia in rats [58]. TGF-β_1 does not appear to alter CBF [56]. In addition to direct cytoprotection, mechanisms of TGF-β_1 reduction in infarct volume may include effects on circulating leukocytes [57].

Insulin-Like Growth Factors

IGF-1 and -2 are structurally-related 7.6- and 7.4-kD polypeptides, respectively [41, 53]. Each binds to a specific high-affinity tyrosine kinase receptor (IGF-1R and -2R, respectively). In addition, six IGF binding proteins (IGFBPs) are found. In vitro, IGF-1 and -2 protect embryonic rat hippocampal and septal neurons against hypoglycemia and protect embryonic rat hippocampal and human cortical neurons against iron-induced free radical damage [19, 59].

IGF-1, in particular, has been studied as a treatment for cerebral ischemia. Intraventricular infusion of IGF-1 (50 μg/day × 7 days) in mature rats reduces neuronal loss in hippocampus following transient forebrain ischemia [60], although other studies using a lower dose of IGF-1 (2 μg as a single injection) failed to show this effect [61]. Interestingly, protection was lost at the higher dose of IGF-1 when rats were starved prior to ischemia [62]. In fetal sheep, protection against neuronal loss in cortex, striatum, and hippocampus was obtained at doses of 1.0 > 0.1 μg, but not at 10 μg of IGF-1 delivered intraventricularly at 2 h after the onset of global forebrain ischemia, providing a 'U-shaped' dose-response curve [63]. IGF-1 also reduced postischemic seizures and edema at these doses. In models of focal hypoxia/ischemia produced by occlusion of the CCA and temporary exposure to a low oxygen environment, intraventricular IGF-1 (5–50 μg) at 1 h before or 2 h after ischemia reduced the infarction rate as well as neuronal loss in cortex, striatum, and hippocampus [64, 65].

In summary, considerable current evidence provides 'proof of principle' that members of several neurotrophic growth factors can protect brain tissue in experimental models of both global and focal cerebral ischemia. The relatively low doses of growth factors used in the above studies reflects the fact that cells possess high-affinity receptors for these molecules, which amplify their effects through signal transduction pathways. In most of the preclinical studies cited above, growth factors have been administered directly to the brain by intraventricular or intracisternal injection. However, in recent preclinical studies, at least one trophic factor, bFGF, has been delivered systemically. In these studies, intraperitoneal or intravenous bFGF was found to cross the damaged BBB and to decrease the extent of cerebral injury [23, 27].

Based on the promising preclinical data obtained with bFGF, a human clinical safety trial of this factor for the treatment of acute stroke has recently begun at seven US medical centers. This trial is a randomized, placebo-controlled, dose-escalation study of intravenous bFGF treatment in patients having suffered acute thromboembolic supratentorial cerebral infarction within the previous 12 h. Extensive safety data will be obtained, as well as efficacy data using standard neurological and functional rating scales, and diffusion/perfusion MRI scanning [66]. Because growth factors may work through several mechanisms to antagonize cell death after ischemia, it is conceivable that these factors will find a useful role as sole or adjunct treatments for acute stroke. Moreover, because of their effects in promoting neuronal outgrowth and synapse formation, trophic growth factors may also represent treatments that enhance functional recovery after chronic stroke.

References

1 Sabel BA, Vantini G, Finklestein SP: The role of neurotrophic factors in the treatment of neurological disorders; in Vecsei L, Freese A, Schwartz KJ, Beal MF (eds): Neurological Disorders: Novel Experimental and Therapeutic Strategies. New York, Ellis Horwood, 1992, pp 113–180.

2 Mattson MP, Scheff SW: Endogenous neuroprotection factors and traumatic brain injury: Mechanisms of action and implications for therapy. J Neurotrauma 1994;11:3–33.

3 Mattson MP, Barger SW: Programmed cell life: Neuroprotective signal transduction and ischemic brain injury; in Moskowitz MA, Caplan LR (eds): Cerebrovascular Diseases: The 19th Princeton Stroke Conference. Newton, Butterworth-Heinemann, 1995, pp 271–290.

4 Berlove DJ, Finklestein SP: Growth factors and brain injury; in Moody TW (ed): Growth Factors, Peptides and Receptors. New York, Plenum Press, 1993, pp 137–143.

5 Mattson MP, Lovell MA, Furukawa K, Markesbery WR: Neurotrophic factors attenuate glutamate-induced accumulation of peroxides, elevation of intracellular Ca^{2+} concentration, and neurotoxicity and increase antioxidant enzyme activities in hippocampal neurons. J Neurochem 1995;65:1740–1751.

6 Ginsberg MD, Pulsinelli WA: The ischemic penumbra, injury thresholds, and the therapeutic window for acute stroke. Ann Neurol 1994;36:553–554.

7 Hossmann K-A: Viability thresholds and the penumbra of focal ischemia. Ann Neurol 1994;36: 557–565.

8 Finklestein SP, Young AB: Excitotoxic neuronal disease: Future therapies for epilepsy, stroke, and degenerative diseases; in Rosenberg RN (ed): Continuum: Lifelong Learning in Neurology. Minneapolis, American Academy of Neurology, in press.

9 Baird A, Klagsbrun M: The Fibroblast Growth Factor Family. New York, New York Academy of Sciences, 1991.

10 Baird A: Fibroblast growth factors: Activities and significance of non-neurotrophin neurotrophic growth factors. Curr Opin Neurobiol 1994;4:78–86.

11 Caday CG, Klagsbrun M, Fanning PJ, Mirzabegian A, Finklestein SP: Fibroblast growth factor levels in the developing rat brain. Dev Brain Res 1990;52:241–246.

12 Speliotes EK, Caday CG, Do T, Weise J, Kowall NW, Finklestein SP: Increased expression of basic fibroblast growth factor following focal cerebral infarction in the rat. Mol Brain Res 1996;39:31–42.

13 Walicke PA: Basic and acidic fibroblast growth factors have trophic effects on neurons from multiple CNS regions. J Neurosci 1988;8:2618–2627.

14 Mattson MP, Murrain M, Guthrie PB, Kater SB: Fibroblast growth factor and glutamate: Opposing roles in the generation and degeneration of hippocampal neuroarchitecture. J Neurosci 1989;9: 3728–3740.

15 Freese A, Finklestein SP, DiFiglia M: Basic fibroblast growth factor protects striatal neurons in vitro from NMDA-receptor mediated excitotoxicity. Brain Res 1992;575:351–355.

16 Finklestein SP, Kemmou A, Caday CG, Berlove DJ: Basic fibroblast growth factor protects cerebrocortical neurons against excitatory amino acid toxicity in vitro. Stroke 1993;24(suppl I):141–143.

17 Cheng B, Mattson MP: NGF and bFGF protect rat hippocampal and human cortical neurons against hypoglycemic damage by stabilizing calcium homeostasis. Neuron 1991;7:1–20.

18 Maise K, Boccone L: Neuroprotection by peptide growth factors against anoxia and nitric oxide toxicity requires modulation of protein kinase C. J Cereb Blood Flow Metab 1995;15:440–449.

19 Zhang Y, Tatsuno T, Carney JM, Mattson MP: Basic FGF, NGF, and IGFs protect hippocampal and cortical neurons against iron-induced degeneration. J Cereb Blood Flow Metab 1993;13:378–388.

20 Mattson MP, Kumar KN, Wang H, Cheng B, Michaelis EK: Basic FGF regulates the expression of a functional 71-kD NMDA receptor protein that mediates calcium influx and neurotoxicity in hippocampal neurons. J Neurosci 1993;13:4575–4588.

21 Rosenblatt S, Irikura K, Caday CG, Finklestein SP, Moskowitz MA: Basic fibroblast growth factor dilates rat pial arterioles. J Cereb Blood Flow Metab 1994;14:70–74.

22 Regli L, Anderson RE, Meyer FB: Basic fibroblast growth factor increases cortical blood flow in vivo. Brain Res 1994;665:155–157.

23 Nozaki K, Finklestein SP, Beal MF: Basic fibroblast growth factor protects against hypoxia-ischemia and NMDA neurotoxicity in neonatal rats. J Cereb Blood Flow Metab 1993;13:221–228.

24 Nozaki K, Finklestein SP, Beal MF: Delayed administration of basic fibroblast growth factor protects against NMDA neurotoxicity in neonatal rats. Eur J Pharmacol 1993;232:295–297.

25 Kirschner P, Henshaw R, Weise J, Trubetskoy V, Finklestein SP, Schulz JB, Beal MF: Basic fibroblast growth factor protects against excitotoxicity and chemical hypoxia in both neonatal and adult rats. J Cereb Blood Flow Metab 1995;15:619–623.

26 Koketsu N, Berlove DJ, Moskowitz MA, Kowall NW, Caday CG, Finklestein SP: Pretreatment with intraventricular basic fibroblast growth factor decreases infarct size following focal cerebral ischemia in rats. Ann Neurol 1994;35:451–457.

27 Fisher M, Meadows M-E, Do T, Weise J, Trubetskoy V, Charette M, Finklestein SP: Delayed treatment with intravenous basic fibroblast growth factor reduces infarct size following permanent focal cerebral ischemia in rats. J Cereb Blood Flow Metab 1995;15:953–959.

28 Jiang N, Finklestein SP, Do T, Caday CG, Charette M, Chopp M: Delayed intravenous administration of basic fibroblast growth factor reduces infarct volume in a model of focal cerebral ischemia/reperfusion in the rat. J Neurol Sci 1996;139:173–179.

29 Chen K, Finklestein SP: Dose-dependent effects of intravenous basic fibroblast growth factor on infarct volume and regional cerebral blood flow following focal cerebral ischemia in the rat (submitted).

30 Tanaka R, Miyasaka Y, Yada K, Ohwada T, Kameya T: Basic fibroblast growth factor increases regional cerebral blood flow and reduces infarct size after experimental ischemia in a rat model. Stroke 1995;26:2154–2159.

31 Bethel A, Kirsch JR, Koehler RC, Finklestein SP, Traystman RJ: Intravenous basic fibroblast growth factor decreases brain injury resulting from focal ischemia in cats. Stroke 1997;28:609–615.

32 Cuevas P, Carceller F, Ortega S, Zazo M, Nieto I, Gimenez-Gallego G: Hypotensive activity of fibroblast growth factor. Science 1991;254:1208–1210.

33 Huang Z, Chen K, Huang PL, Finklestein SP, Moskowitz MA: Basic fibroblast growth factor ameliorates focal ischemic injury in type III NOS deficient mice by rCBF-independent mechanisms (submitted).

34 Stroemer RP, Kent TA, Hulsebosch CE: Neocortical neural sprouting, synaptogenesis, and behavioral recovery after neocortical infarction in rats. Stroke 1995;26:2135–2144.

35 Jones TA, Schallert T: Use-dependent growth of pyramidal neurons after neocortical damage. J Neurosci 1994;14:2140–2152.

36 Kawamata T, Alexis NE, Dietrich WD, Finklestein SP: Intracisternal basic fibroblast growth factor enhances behavioral recovery following focal cerebral infarction in the rat. J Cereb Blood Flow Metab 1996;16:542–547.

37 Yamada K, Kinoshita A, Kohmura E, Sakaguchi T, Taguchi J, Kataoka K, Hayakawa T: Basic fibroblast growth factor prevents thalamic degeneration after cortical infarction. J Cereb Blood Flow Metab 1991;11:472–478.

38 Sasaki K, Oomura Y, Suzuki K, Hanai K, Yagi H: Acidic fibroblast growth factor prevents death of hippocampal CA1 pyramidal cells following ischemia. Neurochem Int 1992;21:397–402.

39 MacMillan V, Walton-Roche K, Davis J: Acidic fibroblast growth factor infusion reduces ischemic CA1 hippocampal damage in the gerbil. Can J Neurol Sci 1993;20:37–40.

40 Figueiredo BC, Piccardo P, Maysinger D, Clarke PB, Cuello AC: Effects of acidic fibroblast growth factor on cholinergic neurons of nucleus basalis magnocellularis and in a spatial memory task following cortical devascularization. Neuroscience 1993;56:955–963.

41 Loughlin SE, Fallon JH: Neurotrophic Factors. San Diego, Academic Press, 1993.

42 Boniece IR, Wagner JA: Growth factors protect PC12 cells against ischemia by a mechanism that is independent of PKA, PKC, and protein synthesis. J Neurosci 1993;13:4220–4228.

43 Jackson GR, Werrbach-Perez K, Ezell EL, Post JFM, Perez-Polo JR: Nerve growth factor effects on pyridine nucleotides after oxidant injury of rat pheochromocytoma cells.. Brain Res 1992;592: 239–248.

44 Shigeno T, Mima T, Takakura K, Graham DI, Kato G, Hashimoto Y, Furukawa S: Amelioration of delayed neuronal death in the hippocampus by nerve growth factor. J Neurosci 1991;11:2914–2919.

45 Tanaka K, Tsukahara T, hashimoto N, Ogata N, Yonekawa Y, Kimura T, Taniguchi T: Effect of nerve growth factor on delayed neuronal death after cerebral ischemia. Acta Neurochir 1994;129:64–71.

46 Beck T, Wree A, Sauer DD: Chronic infusion of nerve growth factor does not rescue pyramidal cells after transient forebrain ischemia in the rat. Neurosci Lett 1992;135:252–254.
47 Lee TH, Abe K, Aoki M, Nakamura M, Kogure K, Itoyama Y: The protective effect of *L*-threo-3,4-dihydroxyphenylserine on ischemic hippocampal neuronal death in gerbils. Stroke 1994;25:1425–1431.
48 Pechan PA, Yoshida T, Panahian N, Moskowitz MA, Breakefield XO: Genetically modified fibroblasts producing NGF protect hippocampal neurons after ischemia in the rat. Neuroreport 1995;6:669–672.
49 Holtzman DM, Sheldon RA, Jaffe W, Cheng Y, Ferriero DM: Nerve growth factor protects the neonatal brain against hypoxic-ischemic injury. Ann Neurol 1996;39:114–122.
50 Cuello AC, Maysinger D, Garofalo L: Trophic factor effects on cholinergic innervation in the cerebral cortex of the adult rat brain. Mol Neurobiol 1992;6:451–461.
51 Liberini P, Pioro EP, Maysinger D, Ervin FR, Cuello AC: Long-term protective effects of human recombinant nerve growth factor and monosialoganglioside GM1 treatment on primate nucleus basalis cholinergic neurons after neocortical infarction. Neuroscience 1993;53:625–637.
52 Beck T, Lindholm D, Castren E, Wree A: Brain-derived neurotrophic factor protects against ischemic cell damage in rat hippocampus. J Cereb Blood Flow Metab 1994;14:689–692.
53 Ibelgaufts H: Dictionary of Cytokines. New York, VCH Publishers, 1995.
54 Prehn JH, Backhauss C, Krieglstein J: Transforming growth factor-beta-1 prevents glutamate neurotoxicity in rat neocortical cultures and protects mouse neocortex from ischemic injury in vivo. J Cereb Blood Flow Metab 1993;13:521–525.
55 Henrich-Noack P, Prehn JH, Krieglestein J: Neuroprotective effects of TGF-beta-1. J Neural Transm Suppl 1994;43:33–45.
56 Gross CE, Bednar MM, Howard DB, Sporn MB: TGF-β_1 reduces infarct size following experimental cerebral ischemia. Stroke 1993;24:558–562.
57 Gross CE, Howard DB, Dooley RH, Raymond SJ, Fuller S, Bednar MM: TGF-beta-1 post-treatment in a rabbit model of cerebral ischemia. Neurol Res 1994;16:465–470.
58 McNeill H, Williams C, Guan J, Dragunow M, Lawlor P, Sirimanne E, Nikolics K, Gluckman P: Neuronal rescue with transforming growth factor-beta-1 after hypoxic-ischemic brain injury. Neuroreport 1994;5:901–904.
59 Cheng B, Mattson MP: IGF-I and IGF-II protect cultured hippocampal and septal neurons against calcium-mediated hypoglycemic damage. J Neurosci 1992;12:1558–1566.
60 Zhu CZ, Auer RN: Intraventricular administration of insulin and IGF-1 in transient forebrain ischemia. J Cereb Blood Flow Metab 1994;14:237–242.
61 Bergstedt K, Wieloch T: Changes in insulin-like growth factor 1 receptor density after transient cerebral ischemia in the rat. Lack of protection against ischemic brain damage following injection of insulin-like growth factor 1. J Cereb Blood Flow Metab 1993;13:895–898.
62 Zhu CZ, Auer RN: Centrally administered insulin and IGF-1 in transient forebrain ischaemia in fasted rats. Neurol Res 1994;16:116–120.
63 Johnston BM, Mallard EC, Williams CE, Gluckman PD: Insulin-like growth factor-1 is a potent neuronal rescue agent after hypoxic-ischemic injury in fetal lambs. J Clin Invest 1996;97:300–308.
64 Gluckman P, Klempt N, Guan J, Mallard C, Sirimanne E, Dragunow M, Klempt M, Singh K, Williams C, Nikolics K: A role for IGF-1 in the rescue of CNS neurons following hypoxic-ischemic injury. Biochem Biophys Res Commun 1992;182:593–599.
65 Guan J, Williams C, Gunning M, Mallard C, Gluckman P: The effects of IGF-1 treatment after hypoxic-ischemic brain injury in adult rats. J Cereb Blood Flow Metab 1993;13:609–616.
66 Sorensen AG, Buonanno FS, Schwamm L, Lev MH, Huang-Hellinger FR, Reese TR, Weisskoff RM, Finklestein S, Davis TL, Gonzales RG, Rosen BR, Koroshetz WJ: Accuracy of diffusion and perfusion MR imaging in diagnosis of stroke. Radiology 1996;199:391–401.

Dr. Seth Finklestein, CNS Growth Factor Research Laboratory,
Warren 408, Massachusetts General Hospital, Boston, MA 02114 (USA)

New Drug Development

Hsu CY (ed): Ischemic Stroke: From Basic Mechanisms to New Drug Development.
Monogr Clin Neurosci. Basel, Karger, 1998, vol 16, pp 128–138

Current Status of New Drug Development for Ischemic Stroke

Justin A. Zivin

Department of Neurosciences, University of California at San Diego School of Medicine, La Jolla, Calif., USA

Tissue plasminogen activator (tPA) has now been proven to be an effective treatment for acute stroke. This result will have substantial impacts on future clinical trials. The purpose of this chapter is to review the main points of the thrombolytic therapy trials and discuss their implications.

Thrombolysis Trials

After considerable development and extensive phase I and II studies, the results of two large phase III studies have recently been reported. The European Cooperative Acute Stroke Study (ECASS) [1] was prospective, multicenter, double-blind, and placebo-controlled. Six hundred twenty patients with moderate to severe neurologic deficits were entered into trial. The entry criteria specified that the initial CT scans should lack evidence of hemorrhage or large infarction. Patients were randomized to placebo or 1.1mg/kg tPA (alteplase) within 6 h after symptom onset. The primary endpoint, recorded 3 month after each stroke began, was a combination of the Barthel Index, which is a scale measuring activities of daily living, and the modified Rankin Scale, which is a global assessment of neurologic function. Additionally, several secondary endpoints were recorded. Although there was an attempt to enter patients very early, over 80% of the patients were treated between 3 and 6 h after stroke onset.

For the primary intention-to-treat analysis, there was no significant difference between the tPA- and placebo-treated stroke patients. However, before the investigators were unblinded, they found that 109 patients were included despite major protocol violations. Many patients had lesions on their initial CT scans that exceeded the protocol-specified limits. Only patients with relatively minor CT abnormalities should have been entered. When the violations were excluded by an adjudication panel, analysis of the remaining 'target population' revealed a significant difference in favor of the tPA-treated patients for the primary and almost all secondary endpoints. No significant difference in mortality and the overall incidence of intracerebral hemorrhages occurred, but large parenchymatous hemorrhages were about 4 times more frequent in the tPA-treated group.

This study suggests that patients treated 3–6 h after stroke onset with tPA may benefit. It is not clear why so many protocol violations occurred, but it may be difficult for physicians to accurately read the sometimes subtle changes in the CT scans while under severe time pressure and better training may be necessary. The main conclusion of the authors was that they had not proven intravenous thrombolysis is effective for stroke therapy, but exclusion of patients with early CT signs of stroke should yield a positive result.

Subsequently, the National Institute of Neurological Disorders and Stroke rt-PA Stroke Study Group report appeared (hereafter called the NIH tPA trial) [2]. These investigators conducted a randomized, double-blind, placebo-controlled trial of intavenous tPA in a total of 624 patients in the US. They required an initial CT scan free of evidence of hemorrhage. Treatment for 1 h with a total of 0.9 mg/kg (alteplase) had to be initiated within 90 min after symptom onset in half the patients. The other half of the patients were treated 91–180 min after symptoms began. The primary outcome measure was a global statistic (the Wald test) that simultaneously tests for normal or near normal outcomes on the NIH Stroke Scale (a standardized neurological examination), the modified Rankin Scale, the Glasgow Outcome Scale (which is very similar to the Rankin Scale) and the Barthel Index. These examinations were performed 3 months after symptom onset by raters who had not previously seen the patients. Two sequential cohorts of approximately equal size were included in the trial. The first cohort was used to decide whether there was any suggestion of treatment activity 24 h after admission, and the primary hypothesis tested the 3-month post-randomization results in the second cohort.

For the primary hypothesis, the global test odds ratio showed that tPA treatment was significantly better than placebo in the second part of the study (odds ratio of 1.7, $p<0.001$). Additionally, the results of all neurologic rating scales were highly significant for both parts of the study, with about a 50% improvement in relative risk for each scale. Combining both cohorts, symptomatic intracerebral hemorrhages within 36 h after stroke onset increased significantly, from 0.6% in controls to 6.4% in the tPA-treated group. Mortality was not significantly altered by treatment although there was a trend for improved survival in tPA-treated patients. In the combined results, tPA administration produced an absolute increase of 11–13% in the proportion of patients that regained normal neurologic function (about 25% of controls fully recovered).

In addition to the trials of tPA, three studies of other thrombolytic substances recently ended. Streptokinase (SK) is considerably less expensive than tPA, so there was an economic incentive for evaluation of this substance. Preclinical testing suggested intravenous SK would be quite hazardous for stroke therapy, particularly if combined with asprin [3]. Nevertheless, SK was tested and all three trials were prematurely terminated due to hemorrhagic complications.

The Multicenter Acute Stroke Trial-Europe (MAST-E) was a double-blind, placebo-controlled clinical trial of 1,500,000 units of intravenous SK within 6 after symptom onset, conducted in France and the UK. A total of 270 patients had been randomized when the study was stopped by its data-monitoring committee. They found no evidence of efficacy, and the mortality rate at 10 days was significantly higher in the SK-treated group. This was largely due to a symptomatic intracranial hemorrhage rate that was 6 times higher in the SK-treated patients [4, 5].

The Australian Streptokinase Trial (ASK) tested the same dose within 4 h of onset of ischemic strokes [6]. When that trial stopped, 340 patients had been recruited. The death rate in SK-treated patients was twice that of the controls, which was a significant difference ($p < 0.001$). Seventy-two patients had been randomized within 3 h after the strokes began and no similar hazardous trend was observed, but the entire trial was canceled.

The Multicentre Acute Stroke Trial-Italy (MAST-I) was interrupted by its data-monitoring committee [7]. This was a 2×2 factorial trial of 1,500,000 units of SK, 300 mg/day of asprin (ASA) for 10 days, the combination of SK and ASA or placebo. Six hundred twenty-two patients were entered within 6 h after stroke onset when the trial was stopped. There was an excess of SK-treated patients who died within 10 days (odds ratio of 2.7, $p < 0.001$). The difference was particularly pronounced in the SK plus ASA group. Two interpretations of the data were published by participants in the trial. Some of the investigators reported that there was a trend favoring treatment with SK (alone or with ASA) or ASA (alone or with SK) [7]. Overall, there was an insignificant reduction in death plus severe disability 6 months after the strokes. The dissenting investigators [8] wrote that, since the trial was stopped when only 40% of the planned recruitment had been completed, statements concerning favorable outcomes were unjustified.

Several conclusions can be drawn from the results of these thrombolysis trials. tPA reduces neurologic damage when administered within 3 h after stroke onset to patients with CT scans that do not show hemorrhages and who do not have uncontrollable hypertension. All types of ischemic stroke patients were improved by treatment, and the benefits substantially outweighed the risks. The role of tPA in patients who cannot receive treatment within the 3-hour window remains to be established. SK seems to be more dangerous than tPA, especially if therapy is delayed for more than 3 h after stroke onset. Whether SK is effective when administered less than 3 h into a stroke remains to be investigated, but there now appears to be little enthusiasm for conducting such a trial. Thus, the efficacy of at least one treatment for reducing neurologic damage rapidly after stroke onset has been proven.

Although the finding of a specific treatment for acute stroke is gratifying, much remains to be done. The successful completion of these trials proves that it is possible to reduce neurological damage after the onset of ischemia. This proof of concept also provides us with some guidelines for future investigations. Two major areas of improvements are apparent: (1) protocols for future stroke trials can now be further refined and (2) new strategies for the acute treatment of stroke need to be considered.

Protocol Advances

It is now possible to improve the clinical rating scales. There have been many debates about the merits and deficiencies of each of the numerous existing clinical rating scales, but without directly relevant data, it was impossible to settle the arguments. We can now use the results of the tPA trials to truly validate several rating scales for acute stroke studies. In the two tPA studies listed above, four rating scales were employed. The results indicated that no single scale was markedly superior to the others in terms of sensitivity. Therefore, it is possible to simplify future trials by reducing the amount of unnecessary data collection.

The Barthel Index is useful for assessing activities of daily living. It was originally designed to help predict the level of nursing home care a patient might need, and a good score simply shows that a person can ambulate without assistance and take care of basic bodily functions [9]. A patient attaining a perfect score might not be able to return to work and can have, for example, a severe expressive aphasia. The rating is generally made by interviewing a caregiver and specific questions concern such issues as whether the patient can bathe without another person being present or maintains bowel and bladder continence. Thus, it cannot be fully independently verified by an examiner when a patient presents with a stroke. Since some other scales do not suffer from these liabilities and are easier to administer, there is little reason to continue to include this scale in future stroke trials.

The Rankin Scale consists of a simple assessment of global neurologic functioning. It usually has five possible levels: no symptoms, minor symptoms, minor handicap, moderate handicap, or severe handicap. There are simple definitions for each level. The scale is clearly ordinal, it can be assessed very rapidly and inter-rater reliability is high without need for specific training. Although the rating levels are relatively coarse for individual patients, appropriate statistical methods with a sufficiently large sample size produces an efficient outcome measure as proven by the results in both the NIH tPA trial and ECASS.

The Glasgow Outcome Scale is nearly identical to the Rankin Scale except that it includes death as a possible rating. The results in the NIH tPA trial were nearly the same for both scales. Therefore, there is no reason to include both scales in future studies. The Rankin Scale has been more frequently used in stroke studies, so it is reasonable to include the Rankin Scale in preference to the Glasgow Outcome Scale for comparisons among trials.

The NIH Stroke Scale is similar to many rating systems that are essentially simplified neurological examinations. Deficits in several major domains of the clinical examination are included and quantified, usually in four grades. Inter-rater reliability has been extensively evaluated [10, 11], and training methods to improve consistency among examiners have been developed [12]. Even so, several questions have poor inter-rater reliability and there is room for improvement of the scale in this regard. Despite this weakness, the result of the NIH tPA trial showed that the sensitivity of this scale was equal to the others. The major advantage of the NIH Scale is that it samples neurological functions representing most major brain functions and it can be administered in a few minutes by the admitting physician.

I would advocate use of a combination of the NIH Stroke Scale and the Rankin Scales in future trials. The NIH Scale can be used to objectively document the neurological deficits of the patient and screen out those with strokes that are so mild that treatment is unlikely to be able to show appreciable improvement. The Rankin Scale provides a general rating of the patients in a way that is easy for nonspecialists to appreciate, since a one point change on that scale represents a clinically important difference. A level to include death can be readily added to this scale. There are several statistical procedures that can be used to combine the results of these two scales, potentially improving their power. The global test used in the NIH tPA trial is one such method, but did not appreciably improve the results derived from the individual scales.

A second lesson from ECASS and the NIH tPA trial concerns the need to enter patients rapidly after symptom onset. Animal modeling studies of stroke have repeatedly documented the importance of administration of treatment shortly after the initiation of ischemia, but such studies cannot provide an absolute value for the temporal window of opportunity for effective treatment in patients. The NIH tPA trial, with a treatment window of 3 h, resulted in statistically significant improvements in the patients. ECASS, with a window of 6 h, did not result in a significant difference between groups in the intention-to-treat analysis. The authors of ECASS contended that the protocol violations were the main reason for this failure, but it is also possible that ischemic brain cannot often survive for 6 h. There was little overlap in the populations between ECASS and the NIH tPA trial (all of the NIH patients started treatment in less than 3 h after the strokes began, less than 20% of the ECASS patients were treated that fast). Thus, it is possible that a major contributor to the difference in the results was the greater delay in therapy in ECASS. The exact length of time tPA treatment will be both safe and effective remains to be decided, but it is likely to be less than 6 h.

A third important lesson is that it is possible to design acute stroke trials to show neurologic benefit. There have been many controversies concerning such issues as sample size, use of surrogate markers, and patient inclusion criteria in the past. In all previous studies acute treatment trials failed and there have been some pessimists who thought that it was impossible for any acute treatment to be effective. Consequently, the demonstration that efficacy could be found with a reasonable number of patients, using clinical endpoints, and including nearly all stroke subtypes (besides hemorrhages), is an important proof of the hypothesis.

Surrogate markers that can identify potentially useful treatments without a full-scale phase III study are desirable, but the US Food and Drug Administration requires proof of efficacy using relevant outcome measures. This is a reasonable expectation, and drugs will not be approved for sale in the US based solely on surrogate endpoints. The hope is that some sort of imaging technique will be more sensitive and objective than clinical rating scales. MRI or other similar indicators of brain function will probably ultimately be important for assessing stroke patients, but it is not obvious that they will be any more efficient in identifying useful treatments than clinical scales. Furthermore, surrogate endpoints must be calibrated against a clinically valid endpoint, and now we have a standard of comparison for this purpose. Surrogate indicators will undoubtedly first be worked out in animal models, but when ready, trials in stroke patients will be required to prove the validity of each marker.

Most physicians who have been involved in the acute stroke trials have agreed that a relative improvement of at least 20% is needed to make the effort and expense of a new treatment worthwhile. Based on this exception, power analysis indicates a sample size of approximately 300 patients per group is the requirement. The tPA trials showed that such a standard of efficacy is attainable, and therefore, the sample size in many future trials can be expected to remain in this general range.

There had been considerable concern, since strokes are so variable, that no treatment could be proven to be effective unless a fairly homogenous group of patients was included in a trial. The practical effect of excluding many patients from a trial is that it greatly increases the length of time required to complete the study. Alternatively, patients can be stratified into several different groupings, but if that is done, the total number of patients needed substantially increases. Thus, the proof that it is possible to conduct studies in which there are few exclusions or stratification levels means that it should be possible to conclude studies reasonably rapidly.

Future Treatment Strategies

There is need to improve on the results of the tPA studies that have already concluded since less than half the patients returned to their premorbid state and many will not be eligible for thrombolytic therapy. It appears that tPA treatment is effective for the first few hours after symptom onset, but the window of therapeutic efficacy of this therapy needs further refinement. A trial to answer this question is progressing. The results of ECASS suggest that there may be some CT scan signs that predict poor outcomes after tPA therapy. These criteria need to be proven prospectively, and the data from the already completed trials may suggest some additional risk factors that should be evaluated.

Intra-arterial thrombolysis is nearly certain to be a useful additional form of therapy. The reason that intravenous administration was tried first is that this makes it possible to treat the patients rapidly after stroke onset. A phase I trial of duteplase for stroke therapy [13] required angiograms before initiation of therapy, and this added approximately 2 h before treatment could be initiated. Therefore, intravenous tPA is the preferable initial approach. However, in instances where this method fails, it is reasonable to then try intra-arterial thrombolysis. Such studies are now in progress.

There is a consensus that thrombolysis alone will not be the optimal way to treat all patients. Most investigators anticipate that some form of 'cocktail', probably tailored to the individual patient, will be an improvement. There are many strategies that may be successful and several are already being investigated in clinical trials.

A variety of neuroprotective drugs may be beneficial. Glutamate, which is the most common excitatory neurotransmitter in the CNS, is released in excess during ischemia. The general theory [14] is that glutamate excites postsynaptic neurons by stimulating several types of postsynaptic receptors. These receptors, in turn, regulate calcium flux into the cells through channels associated with the receptors. During ischemia, excessive extracellular glutamate causes a pathological influx of calcium into the neurons, which then activates a series of pathological intracellular processes resulting in cell destruction. The N-methyl-*D*-aspartate (NMDA)-type glutamate receptor can be blocked by several drugs, and this may decrease the abnormal calcium influx. There has been extensive preclinical investigation of this idea [15], and several glutamate antagonists have shown considerable promise. However, clinical testing of several drugs in this class ended in failure including dextrorphan, selfotel (CGS-19755), aptiganel (CNS 1102) and eliprodil. Two main problems caused these difficulties. The NMDA antagonists can cause phencyclidine-like side effects, and although these psychotic-like reactions are dose-dependent and reversible, they have limited the doses that some pharmaceutical manufacturers are willing to test. The levels achieved in patients have sometimes been well below the concentrations that are neuroprotective in the animal stroke models. Another toxic side effect of some glutamate antagonists is the formation of neuronal vacuoles [16], which transiently appear when moderate doses of some of these drugs are given. At higher doses, neuronal necrosis occurs. This form of toxicity has limited the doses of drugs and most of the agents that have advanced to clinical trials do not exhibit this phenomenon.

Another class of drugs that may be neuroprotective is free radical scavengers. During ischemia, reducing conditions develop and this can lead to generation of highly reactive oxygen free radicals. Under appropriate circumstances, these compounds can initiate a chain reaction of free radical generation that may destroy cell membranes. The occurrence of this phenomenon during in vivo ischemia has been difficult to prove, but several free radical scavengers have produced neuroprotection in animal models [17]. Phase II investigation of tirilazad (U-70046F) showed that the drug can be safely administered to stroke victims, but two phase III trials for ischemic stroke patients were prematurely terminated when interim analyses revealed it was futile to continue because there was no or very low efficacy.

Reperfusion injury is another problem that may be treatable. This disorder occurs in many organs, including the brain. When blood flow is transiently occluded, tissue damage sometimes continues to develop after flow is restored to the large vessels. In stroke patients, this is generally ascribed to re-thrombosis or edema formation, but the no-reflow phenomenon is well described in animal models [18]. Recent evidence suggests it may be caused by leukocyte activation. During ischemia, CD18 on the surface of activated white cells can bind to the ICAM receptors on microvessel walls. The adhesion of the leukocytes to the endothelium appears to cause small vessel occlusion. Later, transendothelial migration of the white cells results in tissue destruction. Thus, even if reperfusion in the large arteries occurs, the obstruction of the microvasculature and tissue destruction may continue. Several laboratories now have shown that various leukocyte inhibitors prevent the activation process and reduce neurologic damage in stroke models [19–21]. However, clinical trials of ICAM antibody (enlimomab) did not show benefit.

Several additional clinical studies of various drugs for acute stroke treatment are proceeding. Gamma-aminobutyric acid (GABA), which is the primary inhibitory neurotransmitter in mammalian brain, causes increased chloride flux across the post-synaptic membrane, and hyperpolarization. In many ways, these actions counterbalance the physiologic and toxic effects of glutamate. A GABA agonist, clomethiazole [22], has been evaluated for treatment of stroke patients. Results are not currently available. Studies of lubeluzole, a drug that has multiple actions including inhibition of sodium channels, are in progress [23]. The initial phase III clinical trials were inconclusive although there was some indication of benefit, and additional investigations are in progress. Ancrod (pit viper venom), an anticoagulant and fibrinogen-reducing agent that may facilitate thrombolysis, is being studied [24]. Nalmefene, an opioid antagonist, is also being tested. The mechanism of action of this class of drugs in reducing ischemic injury is unclear but it has been shown to be effective in at least one animal model [25]. Older studies of another opioid antagonist, naloxone, were unsuccessful. However, when those trials were conducted, it was thought that it was impossible to recruit patients within the first few hours after stroke onset [26]. Thus, the neurologic damage may have been irreversible before many of the patients received the drug. CDP-choline, a drug that may reduce acute damage and aid in neuronal membrane repair by mechanisms that may include restoration of function [27], is being tested. The results of its first clinical trial are encouraging.

More trials will probably begin soon. Some will evaluate additional drugs of the classes discussed previously, and others will explore new ideas currently being tested in laboratories. Drugs being studied in preclinical models include volume expanders, glutamate antagonists acting on other parts of the receptor (aside from the NMDA-related sites) such as the AMPA antagonists, and neurotrophic factors that may either aid in preserving tissue or promote restoration of function.

Thrombolytic therapy will probably become the standard of care for patients brought to the hospital rapidly after stroke onset. The existence of an effective therapy means that it will no longer be justifiable to conduct placebo-controlled trials. New thrombolytics can be tested directly against tPA, but other drug classes should be evaluated in add-on studies. Since many drugs will be administered in combination with tPA, it will be important to consider possible interactions. Combinations of agents may act synergistically, but it is possible for undesirable interactions to occur. As a consequence, some clinical trials will require inclusion of larger numbers of patients because of the need for stratification depending on whether the patients receive a thrombolytic agent. Conversely, some drugs that are inadequately effective when administered individually may be potentiated by thrombolytic therapy which may facilitate access of the drug to the site of ischemic injury. In those cases, fewer patients will be necessary. The clinical trials of combinations of drugs should be preceded by preclinical tests in stroke models that are capable of identifying interactions. Also, it will be important to design the clinical trials so they can be terminated early if there is either an overwhelming success or if it becomes apparent, during the course of a trial, that further testing will be futile.

This is an exciting time for stroke investigators. After many years of frustration and failure, it is now evident that at least some trials will be successful. Pharmaceutical manufacturers are well aware of this potential as are granting agencies. Most important, we will now have something of proven value to offer our patients, and it is probable that we can make important further improvements.

References

1 Hacke W, Kaste M, Fieschi C, et al: Intravenous thrombolysis with recombinant tissue plasminogen activator for acute hemispheric stroke. JAMA 1995;274:1017–1025.

2 The National Institute of Neurological Disorders and Stroke rt-PA Stroke Study Group: Tissue plasminogen activator for acute ischemic stroke. N Engl J Med 1995;333:1581–1587.

3 Lyden PD, Madden KP, Clark WM, Sasse KC, Zivin JA: Incidence of cerebral hemorrhage after treatment with tissue plasminogen activator or streptokinase following embolic stroke in rabbits. Stroke 1990;21:1589–1593.

4 Hommel M, Boissel JP, Cornu C, et al: Temination of streptokinase in severe acute ischaemic stroke. Lancet 1995;345:57.

5 The Multicenter Acute Stroke Trial – Europe Study Group: Thrombolytic Therapy with streptokinase in acute ischemic stroke. N Engl J Med 1996;335:145–150.

6 Donnan GA, Davis SM, Chambers BR, et al: Trials of streptokinase in severe acute ischaemic stroke. Lancet 1995;345:578–579.

7 Multicenter Acute Stroke Trial-Italy (MAST-I) Group: Randomised controlled trial of streptokinase, aspirin, and combination of both in treatment of acute stroke. Lancet 1995;346:1509–1514.

8 Togoni G, Roncaglioi MC; Dissent: An alternative interpretation of MAST-I. Lancet 1995;346: 1515.

9 Mahoney FT, Barthel DW, Functional evaluation: Barthel Index. Md State Med J 1965;14:61–65.

10 Lyden PD, Lau GT: A critical appraisel of stroke evaluation and rating scales. Stroke 1991;22: 1345–1352

11 de Haan R, Horn J, Limburg M, Van Der Meulen J, Bossuyt P: A comparison of five stroke scales with measures of disability, handicap, and quality of life Stroke 1993;24:1178–1181.

12 Lyden P, Brott T, Tilley B, et al: Improved reliability of the NIH stroke scale using video training. Stroke 1994;25:2220–2226.

13 Del Zoppo GJ, Poeck K, Pessin MS, et al: Recombinant tissue plasminogen activator in acute thrombotic and embolic stroke. Ann Neurol 1992;32:78–86.
14 Olney JW: Glutamate-induced neuronal necrosis in the infant mouse hypothalamus: An electron microscopic study. J Neuropathol Exp Neurol 1971;30:75–90.
15 Choi DW, Hartley DM: Calcium and glutamate-induced cortical neuronal death. Res Publ Assoc Res Ner Ment Dis 1993;71:23–34.
16 Olney JW, Labruyere J, Price M: Pathological changes induced in cerebrocortical neurons by phencyclidine and related drugs. Science 1989;244:1360–1362.
17 Hall ED, Braughler JM, McCall JM: Role of oxygen radicals in stroke: Effects of the 21-aminosteroids (lazaroids). A novel class of antioxidants. Curr Fut Trends Anti-anx Stroke Ther 1990;351–362.
18 Ames AI, Wright LW, Kowada M, Thurston JM, Majno G: Cerebral ischemia. II. The no-reflow phenomenon. Am J Pathol 1968;52:437–447.
19 Clark WM, Madden KP, Rothlein R, Zivin JM: Reduction of central nervous system ischemic injury by monoclonal antibody to intercellular adhesion molecule. J Neurosurg 1991;75:623–627.
20 Zhang RL, Chopp M, Li Y, et al: Anti-ICAM-1 antibody reduces ischemic cell damage after transient middle cerebral artery occlusion in the rat. Neurology 1994;44:1747–1751.
21 Lindsberg PJ, Siren A-L, Feuerstein GZ, Hallenbeck JM: Antagonism of neutrophil adherence in the deteriorating stroke model in rabbits. J Neurosurg 1995;82:269–277.
22 Shuaib A, Ijaz S, Kanthan R: Clomethiazole protects the brain in transient forebrain ischemia when used up to 4 h after the insult. Neurosci Lett 1995;197:109–112.
23 Diener HC, Hacke W, Hennerici M, Radberg J: Lubeluzole in acute ischemic stroke. A double-blind, placebo-controlled phase II trial. Stroke 1996;27:76–81.
24 The Ancrod Stroke Study Investigators: Ancrod for the treatment of acute ischemic brain infection. Stroke 1994;25:1755–1759.
25 Yum SW, Faden AI: Comparison of the neuroprotective effects of the N-methyl-*D*-aspartate antagonist MK–801 and the opiate-receptor antagonist nalmefene in experimental spinal cord ischemia. Arch Neurol 1990;47:277–281.
26 Olinger CP, Adams HP Jr, Brott TG, et al: High-dose intravenous naloxone for the treatment of acute ischemic stroke. Stroke 1990;21:721–725.
27 D'Orlando KJ, Sandage BW Jr: Citicoline (CDP-choline): Mechanisms of action and effects in ischemic brain injury. Neurol Res 1995;17:281–284.

Justin A, Zivin, PhD, UCSD School of Medicine, Department of Neurosciences 0624,
9500 Gilman Drive, La Jolla, CA 92093-0624 (USA)

Hsu CY (ed): Ischemic Stroke: From Basic Mechanisms to New Drug Development.
Monogr Clin Neurosci. Basel, Karger, 1998, vol 16, pp 139–150

New Magnetic Resonance Imaging Techniques for Stroke Diagnosis and Treatment

Marc Fisher[a], *Steven Warach*[b]

Departments of Neurology,
[a] The Medical Center of Central Massachusetts and the University of Massachusetts Medical School, Worcester, Mass., and
[b] Beth Israel Hospital and Harvard Medical School, Boston, Mass., USA

Brain imaging with computerized tomography and standard T2-weighted magnetic resonance imaging (T2WI) are helpful and widely used to acutely evaluate stroke patients. They are useful for detecting the presence of intracerebral hemorrhage early after onset. These imaging modalities are typically normal in the first few hours after ischemic stroke begins or may demonstrate on-specific changes, such as absence of flow voids, subtle tissue swelling or arterial enhancement [1]. Detecting the presence and extent of parenchymal ischemic injury usually takes 6–12 h or longer. The ability of an imaging technology to rapidly identify and quantify ischemic stroke damage could provide much useful information. Diffusion weighted magnetic resonance imaging (DWI) has recently been developed and can demonstrate ischemic brain regions within minutes after stroke begins [2]. Other new magnetic resonance (MR) technologies are also being developed that will provide much useful information to the clinician for evaluating acute stroke patients. Perfusion imaging can be performed with available contrast agents to evaluate perfusion of the brain's microvasculature and to measure relative cerebral blood flow (CBF) and blood volume with appropriate techniques [3]. The performance of diffusion and perfusion imaging in humans is optimally dependent upon the use of ultrafast MR techniques which can acquire images in less than 1 s [4]. Ultrafast MR allows for the rapid acquisition of diffusion and perfusion MRI, avoiding movement artifacts. The clinician involved with the diagnosis and management of stroke patients needs to be aware of these new MR technologies, because they have the potential to markedly alter early diagnostic evaluation.

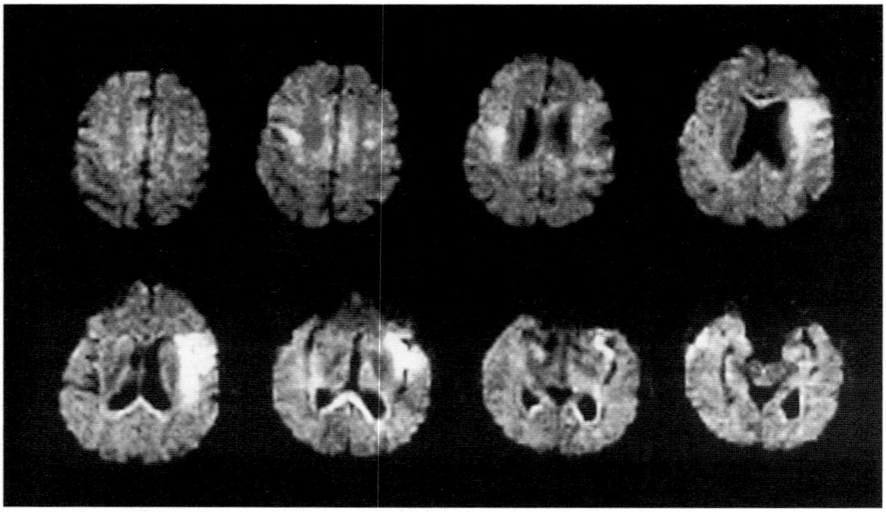

Fig. 1. Multislice DW1 of 3-hour stroke with EPI. Each image was acquired in approximately 100 ms. Acute lesion appears hyperintense (bright).

Diffusion Imaging

With standard T2WI the development of the image is dependent upon proton density, relaxation times and flow. By adding short magnetic field gradient pulses to the standard pulse sequences used to acquire a T2-weighted signal, the MRI signal can be sensitized to the measurement of molecular diffusion [5]. From the DWI images, the apparent diffusion coefficient (ADC) of water protons is calculated as a measure of average water diffusion in m^2/s through brain parenchyma. In normal brains, the ADC values are relatively uniform, but in ischemic regions ADC values rapidly decline. These areas of ADC decline associated with ischemia appear hyperintense in DWI (fig. 1). The cause of this ADC decline in ischemic regions has not been definitively established. The two leading hypotheses are cytotoxic edema through the rapid accumulation of intracellular water, or, alternatively, a decline in membrane permeability to water movement. With both hypotheses, water protons would have less movement over time, leading to an ADC reduction. The ADC decline reflects failure of high-energy metabolism secondary to ischemia, causing membrane pump failure and loss of ion homeostasis.

DWI was initially developed in animal stroke models. The group at UCSF headed by Moseley [2] demonstrated that DWI could detect hyperintense, ischemic regions in cats within 45 min after arterial occlusion, a time when T2WI was normal. In another experiment in rats, they observed hyperintense areas in the ischemic hemisphere as early as 14 min after arterial occlusion [6]. With reperfusion, after 33 min of temporary occlusion, they observed hyperintense regions reverted to normal after flow returned. Minematsu et al. [7], using the same rat stroke model, demonstrated the DWI hyperintense areas observed 30 min after stroke onset are highly correlated with infarct areas determined at postmortem after 24 h of permanent arterial occlusion. Thus, in animal stroke models, DWI detects ischemic regions within minutes after stroke onset and is highly predictive of ultimate infarction, if no intervention is employed. Investigators have determined that changes on DWI correlate with declining cerebral Tesla blood flow, demonstrating the DWI hypersintensity does not appear in gerbils until CBF declined to below 15–20 ml/100 g/min [8]. Interestingly, this level of CBF decline is associated with high-energy metabolism failure and loss of cellular ion homeostasis, supporting the concept that DWI changes with ischemia reflect cellular injury. Further support comes from the observation that ouabain, an inhibitor of sodium and potassium transport, rapidly produces DWI hyperintensity in relationship to its concentration [9]. Ouabain induces intracellular sodium and water accumulation, suggesting that ADC decline and DWI hyperintensity reflect intracellular water accumulation. Glutamate and NMDA infusion also produce ADC declines and DWI hyperintensity. These molecules activate receptor-mediated channels, leading to intracellular sodium, calcium and water accumulation. All of these studies suggest that DWI hyperintense changes reflect cellular changes associated with ischemic injury.

Initial successes in perfusion and diffusion imaging of acute human stroke were accomplished on conventional clinical scanners at 1.5 T [10, 11]. These studies were limited to only one imaging slice and many scans had to be discarded because of patient head motion. This is particularly a problem for diffusion-weighted MRI which are useless if even slight head movements occur. These problems have been overcome using echo planar imaging (EPI), an imaging strategy that permits ultrafast whole-brain imaging.

EPI is a novel class of MRI pulse sequences which can produce image slices on the order of 50–100 ms, and scans of the entire brain in 1–2 s [12]. With EPI, an entire image is acquired from a single radiofrequency pulse. The ultrafast imaging times achieved by EPI are made possible by special hardware that at present have only limited availability. In the next year, scanning equipment with EPI capability will become more widely commercially available and perfusion and diffusion imaging will become available on a more routine basis.

Multislice whole-brain diffusion and perfusion images with EPI can be rapidly acquired, thus the addition of these scans will not excessively prolong

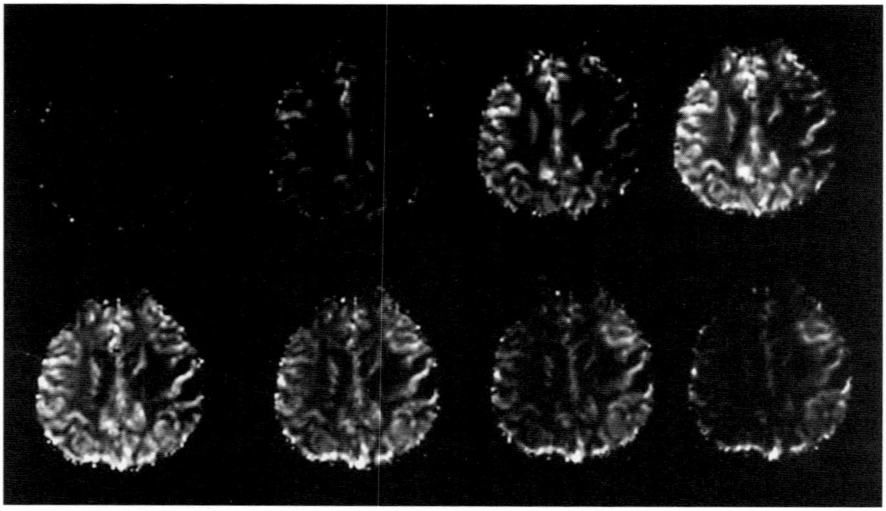

Fig. 2. Dynamic perfusion imaging using Gd bolus tracking. Patients had a 2-hour left middle cerebral artery occlusion. Each image acquired every 2 s after injection of Gd depicts relative CBVs during the passage of Gd. Ischemic territory shows delayed inflow and clearance in the left middle cerebral artery territory with a central core that is completely ischemic.

the patient's workup, nor significantly delay the initiation of pharmacological therapies [13]. With this strategy the ischemic penumbra of an acute stroke can be identified and followed over time. These studies showing perfusion abnormalities that exceed the lesion as outlined on the diffusion-weighted images have provided evidence that the therapeutic window of opportunity in acute stroke in some cases may persist long after the generally accepted 6-hour therapeutic window: lesions evolve within the area of poor perfusion without the development of new deficits (fig. 2). It is also possible to measure the entire volume of ischemic injury to measure the neuroprotective effect of drugs on the brain.

These techniques have the potential to differentiate brain regions that will recover function from those that will result in permanent deficits. Warach et al. [14] studied 19 patients with severe clinical deficits attributable to cerebral ischemia of no greater than 18 h in duration. Conventional and functional (i.e., perfusion and diffusion) MRI scans were evaluated as showing either no lesion sufficient to explain the clinical deficits or a lesion partially or fully explanatory. Clinical outcome was comparably categorized as complete or near complete recovery, substantial improvement but with disabling deficit, or little or no improvement. When compared to clinical outcome, initial perfusion and diffusion MRI was more accurate than conventional MRI in predicting outcome category:17 or 19 cases (89%) versus 10 of 19 cases (53%; $p=0.0195$ by the sign test). In the subset of patients studied within 6 h from onset, functional MRI was an even better predictor – 11 of 12 versus 4 of 12 ($p=0.008$ by the sign test). In conclusion, perfusion and diffusion MRI were highly accurate in differentiating patients with severe neurologic deficits who will improve from those who will not. These tests may have a role in the initial screening and selection of patients with stroke for acute pharmacologic interventions.

Over the next several years as MRI technology continues to evolve and provide better anatomical and physiological information in shorter times, it is possible that the stroke patient may have the entire imaging workup – from cardiac chambers on up – in a single brief MRI session.

Peri-Infarct Spreading Depolarization (SD)

SD is an electrophysiological phenomenon that was originally observed over 50 years ago and is characterized by a slow propagation of depressed cortical electrical activity that rapidly recovers in normal brain tissue [15]. During SD, potassium ions (K^+) move extracellularly, while sodium (Na^+), calcium (Ca^{2+}), Chloride and water move intracellularly. Blood flow increases and SD can be viewed as an energy-consuming process [16]. SD-like events have been observed during experimental stroke by electrophysiological monitoring and the frequency of SD-like waves is greatest during the early timepoints after stroke onset [17]. It has been suggested that the frequency of SD-like waves influences the development of focal ischemia because the energy consumption induced cannot be compensated for and this helps to push ischemic tissue towards infarction. A good correlation between the number of SD-like episodes and ultimate infarct volume has been demonstrated [18]. This relationship supports the hypothesis that SD-like episodes do have an effect on the evolution of focal brain ischemia.

Peri-infarct SD-like episodes are associated with an increase in blood flow in response to enhanced metabolic demand. Taking advantage of this blood flow change, Gardner-Medwin et al. [19] demonstrated a transient increase in image intensity with T2*-weighted MRI that was localized to the cortex and migrated with a velocity of approximately 3 mm/min in animals subjected to an appropriate stimulus to induce SD. Concomitant electrophysiological monitoring confirmed that depolarization was present at the same time that the MRI changes occurred. Gyngell et al. [20] observed a similar change on DWI in a single animal undergoing a focal ischemia experiment. These observations and others to be described from our laboratory suggest that MRI techniques can be developed that will be able to depict SD noninvasively and to determine the effects of SD on the progression and extent of focal ischemia. This approach to the demonstration of SD could also be applied in humans, as the ultrafast MRI techniques necessary to demonstrate SD are currently available for human use. Additionally, the ability to noninvasively demonstrate SD-like waves in focal ischemia could be exploited to determine if drugs that block naturally occurring or artificially induced SD-like waves have effects on the natural history of focal ischemic lesion development in vivo and the extent of infarction.

To assess the ability of DWI to image SD, the following experiments were done. KCl application or a needle stab to the posterior parietal cortex of anesthetized rats was performed within the bore of the MRI magnet. In the KCl group, saline was initially placed on the cortex and ADC mapping was performed on eight contiguous slices (1.5 mm in thickness), using an EPI technique. After the saline was applied, no change in ADC values was observed. KCl was then applied and the ADC maps again acquired every 30 s for 8.5 min. After the KCl application, the multislice ADC maps demonstrated a decline of ADC in the ipsilateral cortex within 1 min in the cortical region initially exposed to the KCl [21]. Subsequently, the ADC decline spread over the ipsilateral cortex at a speed of 3–4 mm/min and returned to normal values within 1 min. We observed similar spreading ADC changes in rats undergoing permanent middle cerebral artery occlusion and a temporal relationship to a rapid and irreversible increase in the size of the ischemic lesion [22]. These experiments confirm that diffusion MRI can noninvasively detect peri-infarct SDs and that these events contribute to ischemic lesion evolution.

Diffusion Imaging to Evaluate Stroke Therapy

The ability of DWI to quantitatively evaluate ischemic lesions within minutes after stroke onset suggests that it could be used to study in vivo the effects of therapeutic intervention on lesion size. Many animal studies have established that ischemic brain infarction evolves over hours and that salvageable tissue, the penumbra, does exist. Therefore, it is likely that some of the DWI areas of hyperintensity seen initially could be reversible. It is also apparent that the absolute values of ADC change varies within the ischemic region, probably reflecting varing degrees of ischemic injury which then worsen over time. In the earliest intervention study, the San Francisco group gave a calcium-sodium channel modulator to cats 15 min after stroke onset [23]. DWI studies demonstrated smaller hyperintense regions in the treated group, as compared to controls, and this was quantitatively confirmed by postmortem analysis of infarct size. Lo et al. [24] obtained pretreatment, postocclusion DWI studies on a single coronal slice that demonstrated areas of hyperintensity consistent with ischemia. The noncompetitive NMDA antagonist MK-801 reduced ischemic lesion size on subsequent DWI studies. Our group has used DWI to quantitatively evaluate the effects of reperfusion and cytoprotective therapy in a rat middle cerebral artery occlusion model. When animals were mechanically reperfused after 1 h of temporary arterial occlusion, a 55% ($p < 0.02$) reduction in DWI lesion was observed when pre- and post-reperfusion DWI studies were compared [25]. With 2 h of temporary arterial occlusion, a small nonsignificant reduction of DWI lesion size was observed. This study demonstrates that the time window for successful reperfusion to reduce lesion size in rats is between 1 and 2 h in this model, and confirms the hypothesis that early DWI hyperintense lesions are, in part, reversible.

In another experiment, we gave the noncompetitive NMDA antagonist, CNS-1102, to rats for 165 min, beginning 15 min after arterial occlusion [26]. DWI studies at 30 and 180 min after stroke onset demonstrated hyperintense lesions which were approximately 70% smaller in the treated group than in controls. Analysis of postmortem infarction confirmed these in vivo treatments' effects. In a second study, the effects of combining reperfusion and cytoprotective therapy was evaluated [27]. The rats received CNS-1102 or saline beginning 15 min after arterial occlusion, and DWI again demonstrated significantly smaller ischemic lesions in the treated group. Both groups were reperfused after 3 h of temporary arterial occlusion, and their infusions were stopped. In the saline group, the large DWI lesions slightly increased, while in the CNS-1102 group a further significant 29% reduction in lesion size was observed ($p < 0.01$). Postmortem infarct size reflected these in vivo DWI results. In an experiment with the glycine site antagonist, ZD 9379, initiated 30 min after permanent middle cerebral artery occlusion, we observed a delayed reduction of ischemic lesion volume beginning at 3.5 h after stroke onset [28]. Additionally, a significant improvement of ADC values only occurred in the penumbral zone in the parietal cortex and not in the ischemic core. These studies reveal how DWI can be used to confirm and follow in vivo the effects of various treatments that can reduce ischemic lesion size. Additionally, DWI can be used to differentiate the contribution of each therapeutic modality, when more than one is employed. DWI could be used in human stroke trials to investigate the effects of a therapeutic intervention on ischemic lesion size. Thus, for the first time, investigators could directly determine if a stroke therapy reduces the size of an ischemic stroke. If the efficacy of a drug in improving neurological outcome is presumed to be related to reducing lesion size, then this information would be invaluable. Additionally, drug efficacy could probably be screened in a much smaller cohort than if clinical outcome criteria were the sole trial endpoint.

Perfusion Imaging

With perfusion imaging (PI), the status of the brain's microvasculature can be evaluated. PI can be performed by following diffusible tracers, such as ^{19}F or ^{17}O, using a tracer kinetic model as is done with ^{133}Xe inhalation and the ^{15}O positron emission tomography method for CBF measurements [29]. These diffusible tracer techniques will not likely be widely used for PI because of relatively limited availability and radiation exposure. The second approach to PI is to inject an intravascular paramagnetic contrast agent, such as those containing gadolinium (Gd) or dysprosium (Dy). At present, only Gd-containing contrast agents are approved for human use. These agents affect gradient echo images which have long echo times, i.e. T2*-weighted images [3]. As Gd or Dy transits through the cerebral vasculature, it locally distorts the magnetic field, causing a loss of image signal intensity (darkening) on T2*-weighted images. Typically the paramagnetic contrast is rapidly infused intravenously and serial T2* images are obtained over seconds to minutes using an ultrafast technique which acquires an image in a few seconds or less. Areas of the brain which are not perfused remain normally intense while perfused regions appear dark, because signal intensity is lost [30]. As the contrast agent exits a perfused region, it returns toward normal intensity. Cerebral blood volume (CBV) can be indirectly measured by quantifying the rate of T2* change over time. Similarly, relative CBF and transit times can also be indirectly calculated.

PI studies have been performed in an animal stroke model and with stroke patients. In animals, areas with reduced perfusion correlate with ischemic regions demonstrated by DWI. In reperfusion experiments, PI has been used to document reduced flow during arterial occlusion and return flow after the vascular occluder has been removed [25]. This documentation is important because the investigator must prove that reperfusion has occurred in a temporary ischemia model, and it obviates the need for an invasive procedure such as angiography or a laser Doppler flow study. Additionally, Minematsu et al. [27] have employed PI to semiquantitatively demonstrate that an NMDA antagonist improved perfusion to an occluded vascular territory in conjunction with DWI studies showing a smaller ischemic lesion. In stroke patients, Warach and co-workers observed that 11 of 15 patients had reduced perfusion in patients with acute cerebral ischemia. They also observed that PI deficits were commonly associated with arterial stenosis or occlusion or MR angiography and that reperfusion and delayed hyperperfusion could be demonstrated. The potential utility of PI for the initial evaluation of stroke patients is obvious. It could provide a quick, relatively noninvasive way to document localized reduced flow and then to evaluate the effect of thrombolytic therapy on restoring flow or not. In combination with DWI, this information would be invaluable for assessing therapeutic response in regard to ischemic lesion size and blood flow characteristics.

PI techniques can also be adapted to perform functional imaging. With neuronal activation both local CBV and CBF increase in response to metabolic demand. These CBV and CBF changes can be measured using PI techniques. A study with visual field stimulation using Gd infusion and EPI has demonstrated the feasibility of functional PI [32]. Another novel and exciting possible way to do functional PI is to use deoxyhemoglobin as an endogenous tracer. Deoxyhemoglobin acts as a paramagnetic agent, similar to Gd on T2*-weighted images [33]. In activated brain regions, CBF increases exceeding oxygen extraction from the blood, inducing a relative increase in the oxygenation of venous blood. The relative decrease in deoxyhemoglobin produces an increase in T2* and enhanced signal intensity in the activated region. With temporary ischemia in cats a rapid increase in deoxyhemoglobin during arterial occlusion has been observed with an overshoot perhaps representing reactive hyperemia after reperfusion [34]. Thus, the deoxyhemoglobin method could provide a noninvasive way to do functional PI and to do PI studies in stroke patients. In the early hours after stroke onset the region of perfusion deficit may be substantially larger than the abnormal diffusion region. This initial mismatch may help to identify ischemic tissue that is potentially reversible with the initiation of thrombolytic and/or neuroprotective therapy.

Conclusion

Major advances of MRI technology for the evaluation of acute ischemic stroke patients are rapidly evolving [35]. With DWI the clinician should be able to see the ischemic regions when the patient initially arrives for neurological evaluation. The location and extent of the ischemic insult should be apparent, confirming the clinical assessment or shedding illumination when precise localization is puzzling. Early DWI lesion detection can also be used as an in vivo marker of therapeutic response. PI provides complimentary information about the circulatory status of the brain. It can also be used to evaluate therapeutic responses, when documenting absent flow and its return is important. These two complimentary MR techniques should provide the clinician with vital information about the mechanism and consequences of focal brain injury.

References

1 Bryan RL, Levy LM, Whitlow WD, Killian JM, Preziosi TJ, Rosario JA: Diagnosis of acute cerebral infarction: Comparison of CT and MR imaging. AJNR 1991;157:585–597.

2 Moseley ME, Kucharczyk J, Mintorovitch J, Cohen Y, Kurmanewicz N, Derugin N, Argari H, Norman D: Diffusion-weighted MR imaging of acute stroke: Correlation of T2-weighted and magnetic susceptibility-enhanced MR imaging in cats. AJNR 1990;11:423–429.

3 Rosen BR, Belliveau JW, Chein D: Perfusion imaging by nuclear magnetic resonance. Magn Reson Q 1989;5:263–281.

4 Stehling MK, Turner R, Mansfield P: Echo planar imaging: Magnetic resonance imaging in a fraction of a second. Science 1991;254:43–50.

5 LeBihan D: Molecular diffusion nuclear magnetic resonance imaging. Magn Reson Q 1991;7:1–30.

6 Mintorovich J, Moseley ME, Chileuih L, Shinuzu C, Cohen Y, Weinstein PR: Comparison of diffusion and T2-weighted MRI for the early detection of cerebral ischemia and reperfusion in rats. Magn Reson Med 1991;18:39–50.

7 Minematsu K, Fisher M, Li L, Sotak CH, Davis MA, Frandaca MS: Diffusion-weighted magnetic resonance imaging: Rapid quantitative detection of focal brain ischemia. Neurology 1992;42:235–240.

8 Busza AL, Allen KL, King MD, Von Bruggen N, Williams SR, Gadian DG: Diffusion-weighted imaging studies of cerebral ischemia in gerbils: Potential relevance to energy failure. Stroke 1992; 23:1602–1613.

9 Benveniste H, Hedlund LW, Johnson GA: Mechanism of detection of acute cerebral ischemia by diffusion-weighted resonance spectroscopy. Stroke 1992;23:746–754.

10 Warach S, Chien D, Li W, Ronthal M, Edelman RR: Rapid diffusion imaging of acute cerebral infarction. Neurology 1992;42:1717–1723.

11 Warach S, Li W, Ronthal M, Edelman RR: Evaluation of acute cerebral ischemia using dynamic contrast-enhanced MR and MR angiography. Radiology 1992;182:41–47.

12 Warach S, Gan J, Siewert B, Wiclopotski P, Edelman RR: Acute human stroke studied by whole brain echo planar diffusion-weighted magnetic resonance imaging. Ann Neurol 1995;37:231–241.

13 Warach S: New magnetic resonance imaging technologies for stroke diagnosis and treatment evaluation; in Fisher M (ed): Stroke Therapy. Boston, Butterworth-Heinemann, 1995, pp 65–80.

14 Warach S, Dashe JF, Edelman RR: Clinical outcome in ischemic stroke predicted by early diffusion-weighted and perfusion magnetic resonance imaging. J Cereb Blood Flow Metab 1996;16:53–59.

15 Leao AAP: Further observations on the spreading depression activity in the cerebral cortex. J Neurophysiol 1947;10:409–414.

16 Lauritzen M: Cerebral blood flow in migraine and cortical spreading depression. Acta Neurol Scand 1976;67(suppl 113):4–40.

17 Nedergaand M, Hansen AJ: Characterization of cortical depolarizations evoked in cerebral ischemia. J Cereb Blood Flow Metab 1993;13:568–575.

18 Gill R, Andine P, Hillercd C, Persson L, Hagberg H: The effect of MK-801 on cortical spreading depression in the penumbral zone following focal ischaemia in the rat. J Cereb Blood Flow Metab 1992;12:371–379.

19 Gardner-Medwin AR, van Bruggen N, Williams SP, Ahier RG: Magnetic resonance imaging of propagating waves of spreading depression in the anesthetized rat. J Cereb Blood Flow Metab 1994; 14:7–11.

20 Gyngell ML, Back TL, Hoehn-Berlage M, Konno K, Hossmann K-A: Transient cell depolarization after permanent middle cerebral artery occlusion: An observation by diffusion-weighted MRI and localized 1H-MRS. Magn Res Med 1994;31:337–341.

21 Hasegawa Y, Latour LL, Formato JE, Sotak CH, Fisher M: Spreading waves of a reduced diffusion coefficient of water in nomral and ischemic rat brain. J Cereb Blood Flow Metab 1995;15:179–187.

22 Takano K, Latour LL, Formato JE, Carano RD, Helvier KL, Haregawa Y, Sotak CM, Fisher M: The role of spreading depression in focal ischemia evaluated by diffusion mapping. Ann Neurol 1996;39:327–337.

23 Kucharczuk J, Minorovitch J, Moseley ME, Derugin N, Norman D: Ischemic brain damage: Reduction by sodium-calcium ion channel modulator RS-87476. Radiology 1991;179:221–227.

24 Lo EH, Matsumoto K, Pierce AR, Garrido L, Luttinger O: Pharmacological reversal of acute diffusion-weighted magnetic resonance imaging in focal cerberal ischemia. J Cereb Blood Flow Metab 1994;14:597–603.
25 Minematsu K, Li L, Sotak CH, Davis MA, Fisher M: Reversible focal ischemic injury demonstrated by diffusion-weighted magnetic resonance imaging. Stroke 1992;23:1304–1311.
26 Minematsu K, Fisher M, Li L, Davis MA, Knapp AG, Cotter RE, McBurney RN, Sotak CH: Effects of a novel NMDA antagonist on experimental stroke rapidly and quantitatively assessed by diffusion-weighted MRI. Neurology 1993;42:397–403.
27 Minematsu K, Fisher M, Li L, Sotak CH: Diffusion and perfusion MRI studies to evaluate a noncompetitive NMDA antagonist and reperfusion in experimental stroke. Stroke 1993;24:2074–2081.
28 Takano K, Formato JE, Tatlsumak T, Carano RAD, Bermann Z, Pullan LVN, Barc TM, Sotak CH, Fisher M: Effects of the glycine antagonist, 20 9379, on experimental focal brain ischemia in rats. (abstract). Stroke 1996;27:123.
29 Nell JJ: The validation of freely diffusible tracer methods with NMR detection for measurement of blood flow. Magn Reson Med 1991;19:299–304.
30 Belliveau JW, Rosen BR, Kantor HL, Rzedzian RR, Kennedy D, Buchbinder RR, Veven TM, Cohen MS, Pykett IL, Brady TJ: Functional cerebral imaging by susceptibility contrast MR. Magn Reson Med 1990;14:538–546.
31 Wendland MF, White DL, Aicher KP, Trnka AA, Boreley ME: Detection with echo-planar MR imaging of transit of susceptibility contrast medium in a rat model of regional brain ischemia. J Magn Reson Imaging 1991;1:285–292.
32 Belliveau JW, Kennedy DW, McKinstry RC, Buchbinder BR, Weisskoff RM, Cohen MS, Vever JM, Brady TJ, Rosen BR: Functional mapping of the human visual cortex by magnetic resonance imaging. Science 1991;254:716–718.
33 Ogawa S, Lee TM, Kay AR, Tank DW: Brain magnetic resonance imaging with contrast dependent on blood oxygenation. Proc Natl Acad Sci USA 1990;87:9868–9872.
34 DeCrespigny AJ, Wendland MF, Derugin N, Kozniewsk E, Moseley ME: Real-time observation of transient focal ischemia and hyperemia in cat brain. Magn Res Med 1992;27:391–397.
35 Fisher M, Prichard JW, Warach S: New magnetic resonance techniques for acute ischemic stroke. JAMA 1995;274:908–911.

Marc Fisher, MD, The Medical Center of Central Massachusetts, 119 Belmont Street, Worcester, MA 01605-2982 (USA)

Addendum

Recent work has demonstrated that a lesion's size on diffusion, perfusion and T2-weighted MRI correlates with clinical severity and outcome. In 50 patients diagnosed with acute ischemic stroke (<24 h) within the middle cerebral artery territory, lesion volume was measured by diffusion-weighted imaging. Thirty-four patients also had volumes measured by T2-weighted imaging chronically (median 7.5 weeks, mean 15.9 weeks). Clinical severity was measured in the acute and chronic stages by the National Institutes of Health Stroke Scale Score (NIHSSS) and the Barthel Index. Volumes of ischemic lesions at acute and chronic timepoints were measured. Acute lesion volumes correlated with the acute NIHSSS ($r = 0.56$, $p < 0.0001$), the chronic

NIHSSS ($r=0.63$, $p<0.0001$), and the chronic lesion volume ($r=0.84$, $p<0.0001$). The chronic volumes correlated with the chronic NIHSSS ($r=0.86$, $p<0.0001$) and inversely with the Barthel Index ($r=0.60$, $p=0.002$). When only cortically based lesions are considered, the correlations are higher particularly relating acute DWI lesion volume ($r=0.61$) and chronic T2WI lesion volume ($r=0.90$) to the chronic NIHSSS. In conclusion, acute ischemic lesion volumes in human stroke, as measured by DWI, correlated with clinical severity and outcome. These results provide evidence that ischemic lesion volumes determined by DWI acutely may be predictive of clinical severity and outcome, and thereby may support a role for DWI in the assessment of acute stroke therapies in clinical trials [1, 2]. Further analysis using combined DWI and volumes of hypoperfusion lesions have demonstrated that the larger volume of diffusion or perfusion abnormality correlates with NIHSSS at 0.90. To determine the frequency and time course with which enlargement of ischemic lesions occurs in human stroke and to study the effect of the state of perfusion on lesion enlargement, acute lesion volumes were determined by DWI and compared to lesion volumes by T2-weighted images at 7 days or later. Forty-four measurements were performed between 2 and 53 h after onset in 28 patients. Thirteen patients also had MRI perfusion imaging performed. In 12/28 patients (43%) the initial lesion volume increased by 20% or greater. Enlargement of the ischemic lesion volume ranged from 12/28 (43%) at >2 h to 10/26 (38%) at >6 h, 4/15 (27%) at >24 h, and 2/6 (33%) at >48 h. In 7/10 patients where the hypoperfusion volume exceeded the volume of DWI abnormality acutely, enlargement of the lesion volume by 20% or greater occurred. This study provides evidence that substantial enlargement of human cerebral ischemic lesion volumes may occur beyond the first 6, 12, or 24 h after onset. A mismatch acutely, between the region of hypoperfusion (larger) and the region of diffusion abnormality (smaller) may be predictive of ischemic lesion enlargement.

References

1 Lovblad KO, Baird AE, Schlaug G, Benfield A, Siewert B, Voetsch B, Connor A, Burzynski C, Edelman RR, Warach S: Ischemic lesion volumes in acute stroke by diffusion-weighted MRI correlate with clinical outcome. Ann Neurol 1997;42:144–170.

2 Baird AE, Benfield A, Schlaug G, Siewert B, Lovblad KO, Edelman RR, Warach S: Enlargement of human cerebral ischemic lesions measured by diffusion-weighted magnetic resonance imaging. Ann Neurol 1997;41:581–589.

Hsu CY (ed): Ischemic Stroke: From Basic Mechanisms to New Drug Development.
Monogr Clin Neurosci. Basel, Karger, 1998, vol 16, pp 151–162

Future Directions in Research and Development of New Treatments for Ischemic Stroke

Paul T. Akins, Chung Y. Hsu

Cerebrovascular Disease Section, Department of Neurology,
Washington University School of Medicine, St. Louis, Mo., USA

Substantial advances have been made in the last 20 years in the diagnosis and treatment of cerebrovascular disease. The preceding chapters describe our current understanding of the pathophysiology of cerebral ischemia. This foundation has been used to rationally develop and test new therapies designed to reduce brain injury and improve outcome after acute ischemic stroke. In this chapter, we will reflect on the present state of the field and discuss future directions of stroke research and treatment. As physicians who provide care to patients with strokes, we will place emphasis on the clinical application of this research.

Stroke Prevention: Primary and Secondary

The best treatment for stroke is stroke prevention. The major risk factors for stroke such as hypertension, smoking, diabetes, and heart disease have long been identified. Public education has led to important changes in the lifestyle of the community. The diagnosis and treatment of cerebrovascular disease risk factors by primary care physicians likely contributed to the dramatic reductions in the incidence of stroke mortality from 1917 to 1992 in the US [1]. The treatment of hypertension, in particular, may be a major factor behind this reduction [2], although this has been recently questioned [3]. A striking example of the contribution of modifiable risk factors [4, 5] can be seen in the sharp decline in stroke mortality for the Stroke Belt in the southeast region of the US. This area derives its name from the high regional stroke mortality. The largest reduction in stroke mortality was observed in African American men in this region falling from 980/100,000 in 1968 to 400/100,000 in 1991. While this positive step is encouraging, stroke-related deaths in the Stroke Belt remains high compared to other regions. Further research is needed to fully account for the high stroke mortality in these regions. Likewise, the broad range of stroke mortality rates across countries suggests that additional environmental factors may be at work [1].

It is unclear whether the reductions observed in stroke incidence and mortality attributable to a modification of primary risk factors will continue [6]. In recent years, the decline in stroke mortality rate has begun to level off. While the treatments available to treat hypertension, diabetes, and heart disease have advanced, there is ample room for major breakthroughs. In particular, new approaches for insulin-dependent diabetes such as transplantation of islet cells or genetically engineered cells may reduce long-term diabetic complications including stroke. Another area long overdue for effective treatment is obesity. This risk factor is epidemic in the US, but the present treatments of obesity are disappointing. The rapidly appearing reports regarding the biology of leptin [7] provide hope that better treatments for obesity will be forthcoming.

Still the most effective strategies for stroke prevention are to improve the health habits of the community. The massive public education campaigns of the American Heart Association, National Stroke Association, National Institute of Neurological Disorders and Stroke, and other organizations have been extremely valuable in educating the community in the prevention of stroke and heart disease. Stroke neurologists and researchers will need to further increase their level of involvement in community education.

Many epidemiological studies have made it clear that patients who have suffered either strokes or transient ischemic attacks are at high risk for recurrent strokes [8]. Secondary stroke prevention trials have provided strong evidence that these patients can lower their risk for subsequent stroke [9]. Proven treatments include endarterectomy for carotid artery stenosis, antiplatelet therapy with aspirin or ticlopidine, and oral anticoagulation for patients with atrial fibrillation. But many controversies in secondary stroke prevention remain unanswered.

The proper role of oral anticoagulation to prevent strokes (outside the clinical setting of atrial fibrillation) is guaranteed to evoke lively discussion among neurologists. Ongoing stroke prevention studies such as the Warfarin-Aspirin Recurrent Stroke Study will address this issue, but we anticipate the need for future trials to refine this knowledge. For example, the role of anticoagulation in particular clinical settings such as symptomatic intracranial atherosclerosis will require further study.

Despite available effective antiplatelet and anticoagulant agents, advances are needed. The recent results with clopidogrel [10] reconfirm that thienopyridine derivatives are clinically efficacious antiplatelet agents. Notably, the undesirable side effect of neutropenia observed in a small percentage of patients treated with ticlopidine was not observed with clopidogrel. The role of dipyridamole will merit further consideration given the tantalizing result of the European Stroke Prevention Study 2 [11]. This study suggested that combination treatment with low-dose aspirin and dipyridamole provided additive benefits in stroke prevention. Warfarin is a potent anticoagulant, but alternative treatments with more predictable dosing, immediate onset of anticoagulant activity, lower bleeding risks, and less laboratory monitoring would be a major advance. Recent successes using monoclonal antibodies to block the platelet glycoprotein IIB-IIIA complex in the clinical setting of coronary angioplasty may lead to oral agents that act directly on this complex.

The best treatment for extracranial atherosclerosis in carotid and vertebral arteries will continue to evolve. The utility of carotid endarterectomy in selected patients has been demonstrated through well-designed prospective trials. The success of balloon angioplasty and stenting in the treatment of coronary artery disease has increased enthusiasm for carotid and vertebral angioplasty and stenting. The unknown incidence of potential complications such as restenosis, acute occlusions, and cerebral embolizations, however, makes it imperative that this treatment be compared side-to-side with endarterectomy. Already, a clinical trial, the Carotid and Vertebral Artery Transluminal Angioplasty Study, is in progress in Europe, and trials have also been instituted in North America.

Despite the many positive studies in secondary stroke prevention, the available therapeutic strategies remain limited. The medical treatments all work primarily by interfering with clotting. The natural history of the vasculopathies that underlie many strokes is probably unaltered by the current therapies for secondary stroke prevention. In contrast, lipid-lowering agents can halt coronary artery atherosclerosis and even reverse it in some patients [12].

Further research into the basic mechanisms of extracranial and intracranial atherosclerosis may identify novel therapeutic strategies to stabilize or reverse cerebrovascular disease. Cerebral vessels share some features of the pathophysiology of atherosclerosis seen in other organs, but other factors must be involved. For example, the well-established relationship of hyperlipidemia and coronary artery disease does not clearly apply to stroke [13]. Non-atherosclerotic vasculopathies such as sickle cell disease, Moya-Moya, sympathomimetic drug-induced vasculopathy, genetic vasculopathies such as cerebral autosomal dominant arteriopathy with subcortical infarcts and leukoencephalopathy, and dissections, all lead to stroke through poorly characterized mechanisms. These less common diseases may conceal important clues about how cerebral blood vessels respond to injury.

Early Management of Acute Stroke Patients

The discovery of effective treatments for acute stroke will revolutionize the approach to its early diagnosis and treatment. Already, the results of the NINDS iv rt-PA trial [14; Zivin, this volume] have led to accelerated care of patients with acute ischemic stroke in many medical centers. The impressive array of phase-III trials of drugs for acute ischemic stroke, nearing completion, will likely expand treatment options. However, even after effective therapies are identified, a key limiting factor in acute stroke treatment will continue to be the delayed presentation of patients to medical centers after the onset of stroke symptoms. For example, approximately 15,000 patients were screened in recent phase-III intravenous thrombolytic stroke trials to enroll about 600 patients [14, 15]. Many patients were excluded because of late presentation. Ongoing sites in acute stroke clinical trials have been struggling with this problem with some success. Through public awareness and education programs, the median time from stroke onset to emergency room presentation was reduced from 5 h to 2 h and 20 min at one of the centers participating in the NINDS iv rt-PA pilot study [16]. To address stroke education at the national level in the public and medical communities in the US, the Brain Attack Coalition was formulated with broad support from many national health and professional organizations.

The prevailing view regarding acute stroke treatment is that treatment must be instituted within a narrow therapeutic window of 3–6 h. This short interval has been defined through experiments performed in established rodent and primate stroke models. In practice, the clinical diversity encountered in stroke patients may translate into a broader range of therapeutic windows [17]. Most animal models produce ischemia primarily in the cortex and basal ganglia in the territory of the middle cerebral artery. Many patients' strokes, however, arise from small vessel occlusions that lesion white matter tracts for descending motor or ascending sensory pathways. Under normal conditions, white matter has lower blood flow compared to gray matter and may tolerate ischemia longer.

The timing of spontaneous reperfusion may also influence the therapeutic window for an individual patient. Reperfusion was present in about one third of patients studied with position emission tomography within 48 h [18]. However, preliminary data from the Emergency Management of Stroke Bridging Study [19] suggests that the majority of patients with moderate to severe strokes will have arterial occlusions within a 4-hour window. Clinical variability of the circle of Willis and other sources of collateral blood flow also probably contribute to an individual patient's ability to tolerate focal ischemia. Until we have tools that will accurately determine the status of cerebral infarction in an individual patient, the therapeutic window will continue to be a rigidly defined interval.

The neuroimaging tools required to make individualized stroke treatments possible are under development [Fisher and Warach, this volume]. Techniques are needed to rapidly and quantitatively assess the site of vascular occlusion(s), cerebral blood flow, cerebral metabolism, and the extent of reversible and irreversible injury for individual patients at the time of presentation. Such information could guide decisions regarding intravenous or intra-arterial thrombolysis, neuroprotective strategies, and long-term prognosis. For practical reasons, the acquisition and processing times for these techniques must be brief. The methods must be robust enough to compensate for movement artifact commonly encountered in the neurologically impaired patient.

Magnetic resonance imaging (MRI) promises to be well suited for this job [Fisher and Warach, this volume]. Newer scanning technologies such as diffusion-weighted imaging and perfusion imaging make it possible to detect ischemic brain tissue within minutes of stroke onset. Echo planar imaging can rapidly acquire images from patients suffering acute strokes. While current MRI techniques give relative information about blood volume and blood flow, further refinements are needed for quantitative cerebral blood flow measurements. MR spectroscopy may provide complementary data about the biochemical state of the ischemic region. Certain MR signals may serve as markers for irreversible injury. This knowledge would be important if treatments with significant risk for serious complications such as thrombolysis were under consideration. Despite the many advantages of MRI, the sensitivity of this method for detecting intracerebral and subarachnoid hemorrhage may be lower than CT.

The future of invasive neuroradiologic testing in acute stroke patients is more difficult to predict. Local intra-arterial administration of thrombolytic agents has already proven effective in reperfusing acutely occluded vessels [20]. Ongoing trials will address the efficacy of intra-arterial thrombolysis for improving patient outcomes in strokes caused by large vessel occlusions. To justify the additional personnel and specialized equipment required for this technique, it must have substantial advantages over intravenous thrombolysis with similar or lower complication rates. Alternatively, catheter-based methods not reliant on thrombolytic agents could be developed to disrupt and dissolve clots without exposing patients to the risk of intracerebral hemorrhage.

The projected demands for a rapidly mobilized, multi-disciplinary, acute stroke team, on-line neurodiagnostic equipment, interventional neuroradiologists, and specialized stroke units for neurologic monitoring and ongoing treatments may require the institution of 'level-I' acute stroke centers. This is directly analogous to the current treatment of trauma patients with serious and multiple injuries. The creation of 'level-I' acute stroke centers would have a major impact on the role of the emergency management of stroke in rapid stabilization and transport of acute stroke patients. Such centers would be the ideal setting for clinical trials, particularly at the phase-II level of drug development.

While the major 'expenses' of stroke are the lost quality of life, patient independence, and increased need for assistance and supervision, today's health care climate focuses on the monetary expenses required to care for patients with strokes. Currently, there is a shift towards patient care administered by generalists and a bias against specialist-based care. This may not be in the best interest of the patient. For example, stroke units clearly improve outcomes and reduce medical complications in patients with strokes [21–23].

At our institution, Barnes-Jewish Hospital, most stroke patients receive care from the Stroke Management and Rehabilitation Team (SMART). This team consists of the primary care physician, neurologist, stroke nurse specialist, and a dedicated group of therapists, dietitians, and social workers with special interest and training in stroke. Since the introduction of SMART, medical complications from strokes such as aspiration pneumonia and deep vein thrombosis have fallen. Patient and family education and discharge planning are accomplished within the first days of hospitalization. Therefore, the transition to the next stage of stroke recovery, either outpatient or inpatient neurorehabilitation, occurs smoothly. Since the implementation of the SMART program, the length of the acute inpatient stay has fallen by 2 days, and the cost per case has fallen by 15% [Sheedy C, personal commun.]. This amounts to an annual savings of USD 400,000.

The majority of costs of stroke, however, is incurred after the acute hospitalization. Many families give up their jobs and curtail their activities to provide care to family members with strokes. The loss in productivity and independence for the patient and the caregiver is difficult to calculate. Chronic care in skilled nursing facilities is also very expensive. New technologies and treatments that improve outcomes from strokes will likely be translated into reduced long-term costs. Therefore, stroke clinical trials should also track health care costs between treatment groups to confirm this hypothesis.

Mechanisms of Cell Death in Acute Ischemic Stroke

Knowledge of basic mechanisms of tissue injury after cerebral ischemia has led to new drug development [Zivin, this volume]. In all strokes, symptoms arise from inadequate delivery of oxygen and nutrients to meet metabolic demands. Trials with thrombolytic agents and other treatments such as low molecular weight heparinoids and defibrinogenating agents are designed to reverse this initial insult. After the onset of ischemia, a cascade of biochemical changes occurs with multiple pathways of injury. In animal models, many neuroprotective agents have been identified that ameliorate damage after focal cerebral ischemia.

A key early step in the pathway is the excessive release of glutamate leading to excitotoxicity [Choi, this volume]. Several promising agents designed to block excitotoxicity are in phase-III clinical trials, and most act on the N-methyl-*D*-aspartate channel. Previous trials with dextrophan, selfotel, and eliprodil have not demonstrated improved patient outcomes [Zivin, this volume]. Clinical utility of these agents may be limited, since prominent CNS side effects have been noted at doses projected to be therapeutic based on animal data. In animal models, antagonists at non-N-methyl-*D*-aspartate glutamate receptors such as the AMPA receptor may offer additional strategies to block glutamate neurotoxicity. Combined treatment with glutamate antagonists and other therapeutic agents may be synergistic or additive [24–27]. Ion channel blockers for sodium and calcium channels lower metabolic demand and reduce the influx of extracellular calcium level. Most are well tolerated, although calcium channel blockers in particular have the undesirable side effect of lowering blood pressure.

Oxidative stress and the generation of oxygen free radicals cause further injury through several mechanisms including lipid peroxidation and DNA damage [Chan, this volume]. Free radical scavengers reduce the volume of ischemic infarction in animal stroke models and are under clinical investigation. Acute stroke trials with tirilazad, a potent antioxidant, have not demonstrated improved patient outcomes. The role of nitric oxide in ischemic brain injury is complex [Dalkara and Moskowitz, this volume]. Since production of endothelial nitric oxide appears protective and neuronal production may be detrimental, pharmacologic interventions must be selective for the target cell type. The immune system is activated following cerebral ischemia and may augment tissue injury [Zhang and Chopp, this volume]. Antibodies directed against intercellular adhesion molecule-1 (ICAM-1) reduce neutrophil infiltration and infarct volume after focal cerebral ischemia in animal models. A phase-III clinical trial with anti-ICAM-1 antibodies did not show patient benefit. Many trophic factors are expressed following cerebral ischemia [Finklestein, this volume]. We predict that this will be a rich area for clinical investigation and their selected use may be beneficial both early and late after the onset of stroke.

The recent discovery of dual pathways for infarction after cerebral ischemia, namely ischemic necrosis and apoptosis, has major implications for future therapies [Linnik, this volume; 28]. Most current treatments under investigation are directed at tissue injury mediated by ischemic necrosis. The identification of apoptotic death triggered by cerebral ischemia raises many questions. For example, if necrosis is blocked, ischemic regions may still die through the alternative pathway of apoptosis. The therapeutic window may be longer for apoptosis but require a protracted treatment period. As new genes involved in apoptotic cell death appear with the arrival of each monthly journal issue, the interventions available to inhibit apoptosis should expand. The results of recent experiments suggest that combination treatments targeted at both ischemic necrosis and apoptosis may produce large, additive reductions in infarct volume in an animal stroke model [25, 26]. Ischemia itself is known to damage DNA [29, 30], but the clinical significance requires further investigation. DNA injury may activate apoptotic cell death. Damage to genes involved in repair may limit recovery after stroke.

Acute Stroke Clinical Trials

Current acute ischemic stroke trials have evolved from earlier generations. While previous studies frequently enrolled patients up to 48 h after stroke onset, most ongoing trials begin treatment within 3–8 h. Primary and secondary outcomes utilize standardized impairment scales such as the NIH Stroke Scale and outcome measures such as the Modified Rankin Scale and Barthel Index. These outcome measures still leave room for improvement. In particular, they are not very sensitive to change, and inter-relater reliability may be variable. Persistent cognitive problems common after strokes, such as impaired memory or apraxia, are poorly tested with the current scales. At present, infarct volume calculated from CT scans is a secondary endpoint in many trials. Newer MR techniques may be able to identify the ischemic brain region acutely [chapter 9 by Fisher and Warach]. This measurement could be used to calculate the effect of a treatment on reducing the volume of brain 'at risk'.

Basic research into ischemic brain injury has identified many promising approaches to reduce infarct volume and improve functional recovery. The development of several reliable animal stroke models has been pivotal to advances in the field. Numerous agents have been identified that reduce infarct volumes by 40% or greater. Based on these animal data, many promising investigational therapies have advanced to clinical trials in humans. Despite a tremendous expenditure of resources, only one drug (tPA) has been approved for ischemic stroke treatment in the US.

What accounts for the discrepancies between effective treatments in animal stroke models and the lack of efficacy in stroke patients? The overall utility of animal stroke models has been debated [31–34]. While many experimental variables remain, strokes produced using animal models are fairly uniform. Ischemic strokes in patients are highly variable in infarct location, size, associated clinical deficits, and pathophysiology. Co-morbidities and their associated treatments are usually present. Functional recovery following stroke is complex and heavily influenced by cultural and social factors.

The field has benefited from the recent completion of many major clinical stroke trials, even when results were negative. We will comment on a few key lessons learned from these experiences. With thrombolytic therapies, the major risk of treatment, intracerebral hemorrhage, may offset any potential benefit. Stroke duration, severity, and early infarct signs on CT all increase risk of complications of thrombolytic treatment. If the trial design is able to exclude patients at high risk of complications of treatment, then the investigators are more likely to find a benefit to treatment. However, this high-risk group may have the most to gain from such treatment.

Hypotensive side effects of investigational agents may be deleterious during acute stroke and offset potential beneficial actions. In particular, hypotension has been a concern with calcium and sodium channel blockers, streptokinase, and dextrorphan, a glutamate antagonist. Alternatively, agents that promote moderate increases in blood pressure may have an advantage. Core body temperature is another important variable in determining infarct volume in animal models. Even small changes in temperature can lead to significant increases or decreases in size of strokes. For example, the beneficial effects of MK-801 are exaggerated when the core body temperature is not held constant, because MK-801 commonly causes hypothermia in rodents. Conversely, fever can be detrimental. The preliminary results of a clinical trial testing a murine monoclonal antibody to ICAM-1 confirmed that fever is a negative predictor for functional outcome. We anticipate that the results of the next wave of acute stroke trials will be educational, but predict that the pathway from bench to bedside will always be treacherous.

As monotherapies for stroke become available, combination treatment with neuroprotective agents and thrombolytics will require further investigation. For example, a trial investigating combination treatment with lubeluzole and intravenous tPA is underway. The design and funding for trials with multiple treatment arms will be problematic. Already, competition for eligible stroke patients is increasing between ongoing stroke trials. A central organization to coordinate future trials may be needed to serve as a guiding hand for the field [35]. Even now, a strong argument could be made to run trials with a single placebo group and multiple monotherapy treatment arms to reduce the number of control subjects required.

Neurorehabilitation of Acute Ischemic Stroke

The resilience of the nervous system following injury after ischemia is remarkable. Nearly all stroke patients will gain considerable recovery, if they survive the acute and subacute phases of illness. The process is most striking in the first few weeks and months, but accumulating reports have carefully documented slow recovery up to 2–3 years. Following cerebral ischemia, modulation of gene expression for neurotrophic factors and their receptors [chapter 7 by Finklestein] and many other genes has been reported [36]. Functional neuroimaging studies have provided intriguing results suggesting that ipsilateral brain structures can take over for contralateral regions damaged by stroke. The molecular mechanisms responsible for these changes are not well characterized. With improved understanding of the biology of stroke rehabilitation, it is conceivable that the time course for recovery could be compressed, and the degree of recovery could be enhanced.

Conclusion

The field of cerebrovascular disease is rapidly advancing on all fronts. Through better public and medical education, stroke incidence and mortality can be further reduced using available knowledge. The management of patients suffering acute ischemic strokes will become more sophisticated as new treatments are developed. 'Level-I' acute stroke centers may be required to attract and sustain the required specialized personnel and equipment. As effective monotherapies for stroke are identified, second- and third-generation stroke trials will be needed to assess combination treatments. The results of these trials will rely on more objective and quantitative outcome measures supplemented by novel MRI techniques. The ultimate stroke cocktail may include cytoprotective agents, thrombolytics, trophic factors, and agents aimed at apoptotic cell death. After cerebral infarction occurs, both the time course and extent of recovery may be amenable to therapies introduced during the subacute period such as neurotrophic factors.

References

1 Bronner LL, Kanter DS, Manson JE. Primary prevention of stroke. N Engl J Med 1995;333: 1392–1400.

2 Garraway WM, Whisnant JP: The changing pattern of hypertension and the declining incidence of stroke. JAMA 1987;258:214–217.

3 Whisnant JP: Effectiveness versus efficacy of treatment of hypertension for stroke prevention. Neurology 1996;46:301–307.

4 Howard G, Evans GW, Pearce K, Howard VJ, Bell RA, Mayer EJ, Burke GL: Is the Stroke Belt disappearing? Stroke 1995;26:1153–1158.
5 Lanska DJ, Peterson PM: Geographical variation in the decline of stroke mortality in the United States. Stroke 1995;26:1159–1165.
6 Whisnant JP: Changing incidence and mortality rates for stroke. J Stroke Cerebrovasc Dis 1992;2: 42–44.
7 Halaas JL, Gajiwala KS, Maffei M, Cohen SL, Chait BT, Rabinowitz D, Lallone RL, Burley SK, Friedman JM: Weight-reducing effects of the plasma protein encoded by the obese gene. Science 1995;269:543–546.
8 Sacco RL, Wolf PA, Kannel WB, McNamara PM: Survival and recurrence following stroke: The Framingham Study. Stroke 1982;13:290–295.
9 Barnett HJM, Eliasziw M, Meldrum HE: Drugs and surgery in the prevention of ischemic stroke. N Engl J Med 1995;332:238–248.
10 CAPRIE Steering Committee: A randomised, blinded, trial of clopidogrel versus aspirin in patients at risk of ischaemic events (CAPRIE). Lancet 1996;348:1329–1339.
11 Diener HC, Cunha L, Forbes C, Sivenius J, Smets P, Lowenthal A: European Stroke Prevention Study 2. Dipyridamole and acetylsalicylic acid in the secondary prevention of stroke. J Neurol Sci 1996;143:1–13.
12 Blankenhorn DHG, Nessim SA, Johnson RL, Sanmarco ME, Azen SP, Cashin-Hemphill L: Beneficial effects of combined colestipol-niacin therapy on coronary atherosclerosis and coronary venous bypass grafts. JAMA 1987;257:3233–3240.
13 Iso H, Jacobs DR, Wentworth D, Neaton JD, Cohen JD: Serum cholesterol levels and six-year mortality from stroke in 350,997 men screened for the multiple risk factor intervention trial. N Engl J Med 1989;320:904–910.
14 The National Institute of Neurological Disorders and Stroke rt-PA Stroke Study Group: Tissue plasminogen activator for acute ischemic stroke. N Engl J Med 1995;333:1581–1587.
15 Multicentre Acute Stroke Trial-Italy Group: Randomised controlled trial of streptokinase, aspirin, and combination of both in treatment of acute ischaemic stroke. Lancet 1995;346:1509–1514.
16 Barsan WG, Brott TG, Broderick JP, Haley EC, Levy DE, Marler JR: Urgent therapy for acute stroke: Effect of a stroke trial on untreated patients. Stroke 1994;25:2132–2137.
17 Baron JC, von Kummer R, del Zoppo GJ: Treatment of acute ischemic stroke: Challenging the concept of a rigid and universal time window. Stroke 1995;26:2219–2221.
18 Hakim AM, Pokrupa RP, Villaneuva J, Diksic M, Evans AC, Thompson CJ, Meyer E, Yamamoto YL, Feindel WH: The effects of spontaneous reperfusion on metabolic function in early human cerebral infarcts. Ann Neurol 1987;21:279–289.
19 Emergency Management of Stroke Investigators: Combined intra-arterial and intravenous tPA for stroke. Stroke 1997;28:273.
20 del Zoppo GJ, Higashida RT, Furlan AJ, Pessin MS, Gent M, Driscoll RM, and the PROACT Investigators: The Prolyse in Acaute Cerebral Thromboembolism Trial (PROACT): Results of 6 mg dose tier. Stroke 1996;1:164.
21 Indredavik B, Bakke F, Solberg R, Rokseth R, Haaheim LL, Holme I: Benefit of a stroke unit: A randomized controlled trial. Stroke 1991;22:1026–1031.
22 Langhorne P, Williams BO, Gilchrist W, Howie K: Do stroke units save lives? Lancet 1993;342: 395–397.
23 Webb DJ, Fayad PB, Wilbur C, Thomas A, Brass LM: Effects of a specialized team on stroke care: The first two years of the Yale Stroke Program. Stroke 1995;26:1353–1357.
24 Aronowski J, Strong R, Grotta JC: Combined neuroprotective and reperfusion therapy for stroke: Effect of lubeluzole and diaspirin cross-linked hemoglobin in experimental focal ischemia. Stroke 1996;27:1571–1576.
25 Du C, Hu R, Csernansky CA, Hsu CY, Choi DW: Very delayed infarction after mild focal cerebral ischemia: A role for apoptosis. J Cereb Blood Flow Metab 1996;16:195–201.
26 Du C, Hu R, Csernansky CA, Liu XZ, Hsu CY, Choi DW: Additive neuroprotective effects of dextrorphan and cycloheximide in rats subjected to transient focal cerebral ischemia. Brain Res 1996;718:233–236.

27 Onal MZ, Fuhai L, Tatlisumak T, Locke KW, Sandage BW, Fisher M: Synergistic effects of citicoline and MK-801 in temporary experimental focal ischemia in rats. Stroke 1997;28:1060–1065.
28 Johnson EM, Greenlund LJS, Akins PT, Hsu CY: Neuronal apoptosis: Current understanding of molecular mechanisms and potential role in ischemic brain injury. J Neurotrauma 1995;12:843–852.
29 Chopp M, Chan PH, Hsu CY, Cheung ME, Jacobs TP: DNA damage and repair in CNS injury; in National Institute of Neurological Disorders and Stroke Workshop Summary. Stroke 1996;27: 363–369.
30 Liu PK, Hsu CY, Dizdaroglu M, Floyd RA, Kow YW, Karakaya A, Rabow LE, Cui J-K: Damage, repair, and mutagenesis in nuclear genes after mouse forebrain ischemia-reperfusion. J Neurosci 1996;16:6795–6806.
31 Molinari GF: Why model strokes? Stroke 1988;19:1195–1197.
32 Milliken C: Animal stroke model. Stroke 1992;23:795–797.
33 Hsu CY: Criteria for valid preclinical trials using animal stroke models. Stroke 1993;24:633–636.
34 Zivin JA, Grotta JC: Animal stroke models: They are relevant to human disease. Stroke 1990;21: 981–983.
35 Adams RJ, Fisher M, Furlan AJ, del Zoppo G: Acute stroke treatment trials in the United States: Rethinking strategies for success. Stroke 1995;26:2216–2218.
36 Akins PT, Liu PK, Hsu CY: Immediate early gene expression in response to cerebral ischemia: Friend or foe? Stroke 1996;27:1682–1687.
37 Wiebers DO, Adams HP Jr, Whisnant JP: Animal models of stroke: Are they relevant to human disease? Stroke 1990;21:1–3.

Chung Y. Hsu, PhD, Head, Cerebrovascular Disease Section, Department of Neurology,
Washington University School of Medicine, Washington University Medical Center,
Campus Box 8111, 660 S. Euclid Avenue, St. Louis, MO 63110-1093 (USA)

Author Index

Subject Index